Fear Gripped My Heart

Fear Gripped
My Heart

Rachel Cochran Williamson

P & L Publishing
& Literary Services

Dedication

I could dedicate this book to none other than my Lord and Savior, Jesus Christ. Without Him, I would have no hope.

"Now may the God of hope fill you with all joy and peace in believing, that you may abound in hope by the power of the Holy Spirit." - Romans 15:13

Foreword

In William Shakespeare's Macbeth, Malcolm tells Macbeth to try to talk about his pain and suffering. *"Give sorrow words; the grief that does not speak knits up the o-er wrought heart and bids it break."*

Grief, suffering, loss, and troubles are a part of the human experience. Malcolm's words are certainly wise. In this book, Rachel does this very thing. She and Heath give words to their traumatic experience of physical suffering and spiritual pain. They do so honestly and as transparently as anyone you will read to describe the drama and trauma that accidents bring. It is rare to find such helpful material from the daily reality of trauma and grave uncertainty. That is precisely what they do, and the best part is that they honestly wrestle with what God has written in His Word and how they are to live it out in the midst of their suffering.

You will find that as they tell their story, you will see hope for your story. You will experience something rare today, real people in real pain trusting a real God who loves and cares.

Several years ago, in a time of suffering from the loss of my wife in an accident, I, too, had to put words to my grief. It helped me to wrestle with what I knew in my head but so desperately needed my heart to hear and understand.

As you read this book, please remember that these are real people, a real marriage, and real children that allow you to peek into their troubles and reveal how faithful God is in times of trial.

Psalm 46:1-3 says, "God is our refuge and strength, a helper who is always found in times of trouble. Therefore, we will not be afraid, though the earth trembles and the mountains topple into the depths of the seas, though its water roars and foams and the mountains quake with its turmoil. (CSB)
Later in verse 10, the Psalmist says: "Stop fighting, and know that I am God, exalted among the nations, exalted on the earth. The LORD of Armies is with us; the God of Jacob is our stronghold."

The ever-present, I AM God promises not that our lives will not face trouble but that He will be with us, sustain us and provide what we need in and through it all. The Williamsons are living proof of a God who is faithful to them, and He will also be faithful to you.

As you read this real-life story, why not whisper a prayer to God through His Son, Jesus Christ, to minister to you, to draw near to you, to help you face your troubles and pain so that you too can give sorrow words and find in Christ not a broken but a healed and whole heart.

Ed Litton
Pastor, Redemption Church
Mobile, Alabama

Table of Contents

Chapter 1
Fear Gripped My Heart

For the thing I greatly feared has come upon me,
And what I dreaded has happened to me.
Job 3:25

The phone rang. I knew the second I heard his voice that something was wrong.

"Hey, Rach." Heath said to me in a calm, almost chilling voice. "I just wanted you to know there has been an accident. I don't really know what happened, but I wanted you to hear about it from me and I want you to know that I am ok."

"Where are you?" I responded, with an uneasy tone. "Who is there with you? Are you at the hospital?"

"Not yet, but I am going to be," he said.

As fear gripped my heart, I told him not to worry. I reassured him that I would figure out the details and I would see him soon. The phone call from Heath was heavy. Looking back on my recent call log, the conversation lasted less than sixty seconds. There was no fear in Heath's voice, but my heart was racing with the gravity of the situation.

Immediately, I called one of his co-workers to ask questions. "What could be wrong?" I pleaded. "How bad could it be? What should I do now?" I had no idea what was going on. As questions were storming through my mind, I contemplated what type "accident" could have taken place. *Could it have been a car wreck? Could he have fallen from a pole he was climbing? Did a piece of equipment malfunction?*

My mind was clouded with all the possible scenarios. The sudden fear was crippling and had gripped me to the point I could not remember where I was. In those few, brief moments talking to Heath on the phone, I had no idea what "I'm ok" meant. Was he saying he was "ok" for eternity if he died and was at peace with losing his life on earth? Or did he mean he was hurt but not in danger of losing his life?

I was in shock as I left our 6 children. I can still see the tears streaming from their faces. My heart was broken leaving them. They had as many unanswered questions as I had, and we knew very little about what was going on. Honestly, I had no idea when I would be back to get them and they had no idea if they would ever see their daddy again. Neither did I.

Heath's supervisor who was at the scene of the accident, called me back. I asked which hospital Heath would be going to and I can remember his response like it was yesterday. His only words to me were, "The helicopter will be here in just a few minutes and I have heard Sacred Heart in Pensacola." The words pierced me to the core.

As I hung up the phone, my heart was pounding and my mind was cluttered. *What? Sacred Heart in Pensacola? Helicopter…meaning Life Flight?? What does this mean? Is this really happening to me – to us? How is this even possible?? I literally JUST talked to him on the phone.*

The next few hours would change the course of my life forever. As I found myself flustered and grasping for what to do next, the man I loved most was fighting for his life. As his boots were removed, the charred holes in the bottoms of his feet were revealed. The paramedics caring for him could smell the stench of his burning flesh. His heartbeat was far from being in a normal rhythm and there was no telling what damage had been done to his other organs.

Within about half an hour from his accident, he was being prepared for his life-flight helicopter ride. At this point, his end destination was unknown. His life hung in the balance. He was strapped down to the short, small gurney and his head was secured to the top of the board. With a stature of about 6 foot and 3 inches, the squeeze into the helicopter was very tight and awkward. He was rolled to the inside by one of the male nurses also aboard the helicopter, while the other nurse closed them inside and prepared him for take-off.

As the helicopter took flight, numerous thoughts flooded his mind. As he looked past his feet that were touching the glass of the windshield, he could see the sun beginning to approach the horizon. He began to wonder if this would be the last sunset he would ever see.

The flight was long, and they were redirected in air which added to the flight time. Once they arrived at the hospital, his work clothes were cut off of him and thrown into a pile on the floor. The doctors and nurses began to swarm around him. The icy temperature of the emergency room was almost unbearable. He shivered uncontrollably. The tests seemed to last forever. He knew I was coming to see him, but the wait seemed like an eternity.

The next few hours were critical. His situation was unique and very complex. He was at the mercy of the doctors and the knowledge they had. Even though it seemed like hundreds of people around him, he was alone in that ER cubicle.

Shortly after the tests were complete, I made it to the hospital. After waiting to be called back, I stepped around the corner to where he was. With mascara smeared down my face, my tear-stained eyes met his glassy stare. I made it. I made it to see him alive. Even though the reports from the doctors confirmed that this may be the end for him, we were together at last. I absorbed every detail and savored every second.

Chapter 2
Humble Beginnings

Be still before the Lord and wait patiently for him.
Psalm 37:7 (NIV)

It was a much different experience being born and raised in the large city of Mobile, AL, than my children have experienced being raised in a much smaller town. The streets in the neighborhood where I grew up could tell you numerous stories from my childhood, many of which I will choose not to reveal in my writing. They heard me singing at the top of my lungs as I peddled my new 15-speed bicycle up and down the paved roads, from stop sign to stop sign, and around the cul-de-sac that held the community basketball goal. My bike-riding boundaries were specific and I knew exactly how far from the house I could venture out. The freedom of the outdoors did wonders for my soul. Even as a child, I found it difficult to be still, so I never pushed the boundaries for fear of being placed on restriction and confined to the four, boring walls of my house for a full 2 weeks.

As an 8- or 9-year-old child, there was a peace and a calm in my spirit as I walked along the balance beam my daddy built for me. I could deliver a beautiful symphony with words that rhymed and sounded glorious but did not mean a thing. I could sing about nothing for hours. Those songs could tell you the deepest parts of my soul; a reflection of what my heart felt at that moment. It was just relaxing for me. I was in my element, even though I was all alone.

Our yard was clearly defined with a chain link fence. Our German shepherd, Sarah, who protected our property was confined to the space, but I could climb the fence quicker than any of the boys in the neighborhood. One of our neighbors had the perfect football field as his backyard. Even though he had no children of his own, he recognized what a perfect piece of real estate he had and was willing to allow us to enjoy it. We played there, rain or shine and when my mother called me in for supper, chances were good that I was in the middle of a game on that makeshift field.

Growing up in South Alabama, it was usually hot outside, but there was no place we would rather be. Even though I loved to play outside, I also understood that if my mother saw me indoors, it was a good opportunity for me to fold some laundry or improve my ability to wash dishes. Mom called it "Home Ec." Who had ever heard of such a thing and who had time for dishes and laundry? There were plenty of games to be won on the dirt basketball court next door and the blacktop pavement that was calling my name. The sad truth is, however, that I feel the same way about the laundry and the dishes now that I am grown.

It was such a simple time. Our friends were the kids who happened to live close by. Rarely did anyone have spend-the-night company unless they lived out of town. It was an understood rule that we never stepped foot in any house in our neighborhood. We learned that drinking water from the long, green water hose that was nestled between the bushes in the flower bed was a privilege. We also learned if we failed to roll the hose back the way we found it, we would simply thirst for

3 days. The epitome of failure was to leave the water running from the hose after getting a drink. If daddy found it before mom did, there was a chance that whoever left the water running, would need to pick up a part-time job to pay the water bill.

I grew up with a young sister and a younger brother. If you were to ask them, I was bossy, strong-willed and moody. I expected them to do all the things I wanted to do – everyday. Thankfully, we have grown up to be friends and we are able to laugh (most of the time) about the memories of our childhood.

Grocery shopping with mom was a beautiful art that she had mastered. I listened as she calculated aloud each item as it was added to the buggy. She knew within a dime or two exactly what her groceries would total. Occasionally, she would have an extra quarter left over after buying the groceries for the week. This was the highlight of the week because it meant that the kids could take that shiny coin, place it in the drink machine located just outside the store and choose a soda to share. Sometimes we were even allowed to choose one that had caffeine in it. Thus began my obsession with cherry Pepsi.

Mom made the most of everything that she had. She taught me if I wanted or needed something badly enough, I could get it done myself. I am not a painter, but she taught me how to change the color of the walls. I would not consider myself an interior designer, but I watched her beautifully decorate a table for Thanksgiving with random sticks and weeds she clipped out of the yard and a few pumpkins she retrieved from someone's bag they were taking to the Christian Mission. Thus began my love for re-purposing and decorating.

She loved dishes of all kinds. As a very small child, I remember breaking a piece of her grand-mother's light pink, depression glass she displayed on a dish rack in our kitchen. When setting a table, mom taught me to turn all of the plates the same way, because according to her, the presentation of the meal is just as important as the meal itself. Thus began my desire to notice details.

If daddy was home, he would sing to my brother, my sister, and me as we were falling asleep at night. Many times, he would fall asleep before we did, but we loved it. He can sing really well, but I have never heard him sing in front of anyone else. I was introduced to Elvis Presley and Don Williams while I drifted into dreamland. Some of the lyrics to the songs he would sing were questionable at times, but he changed the words and we were none the wiser. Those are such fond memories. There are still times I hear a song on the radio that does not sound exactly right to me and I am reminded that I am hearing the original song as it was recorded, rather than my daddy's rendition of it.

I watched my daddy work swing shifts all my life. When he would work 7 am-3 pm, we could hear his truck turn into the neighborhood while we were playing outside, even though we lived close to a mile from the entrance. The old, black 1980 Chevy pick-up truck that he customized when he bought it brand new took him back and forth to the paper mill week after week. The 3 pm – 11 pm shift meant we could make a pallet on the living room floor and watch the news with mom. Typically, mom fell asleep on the couch, so we watched the Dick Van Dike show or I Love Lucy while we were waiting for Daddy to get home. Our least favorite was the graveyard shift, which was 11 pm to 7 am. Rarely was I awake when he came home from work, but if I was, I could find mom on the couch, snuggled down in a blanket with her Bible open across her lap and a cup of blonde-colored coffee in her hand. Daddy never called into work. He had earned people's respect and everyone around him knew he was a good, honest, hard-working man. I loved the way he smelled when he came home from the mill. He almost always came home dirty, sweaty, and very tired, but he was never afraid of hard work and he was thankful for his job and we knew it. He taught me to work hard, but I learned more through watching his actions than I did through what he said.

Until the 9th grade, I was home-schooled. The public school in our area was lacking and that played a factor in my mom and dad's decision to keep us home. The benefits of that decision were reaped year after year. I was able to develop a relationship with my mom that I could have never had without it and I am thankful for it even to this day. I was also able to spend much more time with my dad because our school days could be flexible around his work schedule. There were many days that daddy would do a devotion with us on a school morning when he was off from work. This simply meant we got to sit on mom and dad's bed, listen to daddy read from the Bible, and tell stories about work or from his childhood, and rarely did we complete our schoolwork for the day. But mom knew what was most important and she made it work. How thankful I am to this day for the positive, loving influence of my parents on my life as a child.

As a high school freshman, I continued my education at a private school about 12 minutes from my house. I rode to school with a friend that lived down the street and mom picked me up every afternoon after practice. I tried out to play basketball and softball for the private school I was attending. I made both teams by the skin of my nose, but I worked hard. I wanted to be good, but I knew that meant I had to put in more time and effort than others did. I played for a very good coach, but he was tough as nails. He pushed us every day without fail. He drew out of us effort and drive that we didn't know we had. It was through him that I learned to dig deep and truly compete. The back of our practice jerseys said "Expect to Win" and we did.

He required that we practice with shirt tails tucked in, no

ankle socks and we were to all match, every day without fail. We were required to run a lap for every minute we were late to practice for any reason and of course, being late would affect our playing time. He set a high standard, but he held us to it. To be less than the standard was unacceptable, and if I came up short of the requirements, that simply meant I needed to work harder to improve. This is where I learned to take pride in myself, to never make excuses, and to work harder than I thought I could. Contrary to what most people believe in our world today, I was taught that everyone should *not* get a trophy because everyone does not *deserve* a trophy. Only the champion – the one who worked the hardest and earned it – should be awarded the prize in the end.

My first "struggle" or "discomfort" in life came as a high school senior, moving to a new city, in a small town, and being the new kid at the "small-town" school. My dad lost his job at International Paper in Mobile, AL, along with over 1,200 other people, 900 of those being hourly-paid workers, when the plant closed down. It was a tragedy that wrecked numerous families, marriages, and individual lives. All of those people began looking for jobs in the same city, with the same set of skills, and there were not enough available jobs to go around. One of my dad's work buddies, who was also his good friend, saw a small 3 x 5 write-up in the Mobile Press-Register about a job opening in Andalusia, AL, a small town that my dad had only been to twice as a teenager. They decided together to pursue the job, even though it was located more than 2 hours away from where we currently lived. We all knew it, but never discussed that commuting to and from Andalusia would be next to impossible, but he needed a job.

I cannot imagine the fear my dad must have had to even consider uprooting his family and taking them away from all they had ever known, but he never showed it. He had a lot of roots that ran deep in that Mobile soil, but he had always been my protector and I was never afraid because I knew he wanted what was best for me. It was not until later that I learned what a solid, faithful woman he had that stood behind him, and even through the questions and uncertainty, she never questioned his leadership. Mom told Daddy that she would go wherever he thought they needed to go and she proved it to him with her constant encouragement. I can remember watching them on their knees together, day in and day out, pleading with the Lord for direction. Through a series of tests and interviews, along with a few additional hurdles, my dad got the job at a power plant in Andalusia, AL. He moved to an apartment so that he could begin working immediately and mom stayed in Mobile with us so we could finish out the school year.

Starting at a new school as a high-school senior, while also being the new kid in a small town, was the hardest year of my life at that point. I had so many feelings that I did not know what to do with them all. I pouted a good bit. I wore scrub pants and a t-shirt with no make-up and a sloppy ponytail to school almost every day. I never really tried to be friendly. Instead, I sulked about not having friends. During that time in my life, I felt like people did not accept me because I was different. I complained about all of the differences of small-town life, and I was in no way lovely, inside or out. BUT… the Lord grew me through the discomfort.

The process was painful, and the journey was long. I eventually found myself at the edge of adulthood at the grand age of 18. My very first car was a dark, charcoal grey 1987 Toyota Camry. It was made of solid steel. I was about 2 months from graduating high school when I got it. It had no A/C and had an occasional knocking noise that I could easily ignore with the windows rolled down and the radio turned up. It was certainly nothing special, but it got me from point A to point B, most of the time.

I ended up playing softball for the local junior college, working part-time as a nanny/cell phone store manager, taking eighteen hours per semester at the college, and umpiring softball games at the county recreational park in the evenings. I foolishly taught myself how to stay so busy, even with wholesome things, that I could bury the hurt deep enough that I could pretend it was not even there. I learned how to save money and to be sure that I was self-sufficient, even though I was still living at home. For this reason, I never dealt with my feelings tied to the traumatic move from Mobile. I reasoned with myself that I had never cared to be still nor relax in the past, so why now? I could work circles around other people my age and I was not afraid to fail at anything. I was confident that if I worked hard enough, I could find a way. So, from that point on, I worked and planned and thought and saved.

Life kept on going. It did not wait for me to work through things, nor did it slow down for me to carefully ease through the bumps in the road. But...I soon found myself more comfortable, making things happen, feeling fulfilled, and learning to love life again.

Chapter 3
Childhood Perfection

Bless the Lord, O my soul; and all that is within me
bless his holy name.
Psalm 103:1

There have been so many times over our lives together that I have wished I could have known Heath, my husband and best friend, as a kid. I imagine him being the quiet kid that never tells stories or jokes, but who is always picked first when teams are made for a kickball game at school. I bet he made pretty good grades, but he never raised his hand to ask the teacher a question, nor did he ask to sharpen his pencil. I would imagine he never asked to go to the bathroom and was never sent to the principal's office. All the teachers wished for their other 29 students to be just like Heath. They thought he was the perfect student. What the teachers did not know, I would assume, was his school notebook was most likely a football playbook. While he was supposed to be working out math problems, he was probably working on a new offensive formation. If I had to guess, he had that playbook, which boasted of numerous plays he had created, in his backpack at all times and he added to it in class daily.

He grew up with an older brother, 2-1/2 years older than he, who was the life of the party. His brother would give you the shirt off his back and he loved to work on things, but he could get a little loud and carried away at times. Because Heath was quiet and mild mannered, he seemed angelic at home as well. Heath certainly made his fair share of mistakes, I am sure, but those mistakes were quietly flown under the radar. He did not want anything loud, flashy or self-promoting. He and his brother were as different as night and day, but they did all the crazy things boys do growing up together.

I remember Heath telling me a story about heading out to meet the school bus when he was in first or second grade. It had rained hard all night and the ditches in front of the house were full of water. Early that morning, Heath and his brother were playing on top of a hill at the edge of the yard waiting on the big, yellow bus. Once they saw it approaching their house, the boys ran towards the road and jumped, attempting to clear the ditch and catch the school bus. In short, only one of the boys made it all the way across. Heath landed right in the middle of the ditch with water standing in it that was knee-high. And what would you have done if this had happened to you? Probably not what Heath did. He went on to school with soaking wet clothes and shoes that still were not dry that afternoon when he got home from school.

The boys had 4-wheelers and go-karts they would ride on their parent's acreage freely. They were driving deep into the woods and through creek bottoms long before they could legally drive a vehicle. They obviously were not fearful of snakes and critters that lived in those woods as I would have been as a child. I feel certain that many things happened in those woods that jeopardized the safety of those young participants, but what happened in the woods, stayed in the woods. There was no need to bother mom and dad with silly details, like broken toes or bleeding noses from a 4-wheeler wreck.

At nearly every family reunion, there is much talk about Heath and the new go-kart he got for Christmas one year. It seemed that he would ride his new toy up and down the long, grass driveway that separated his house from his aunt and uncle's house. They tell stories of listening to Heath sing over the motor of his go-kart without a care in the world. Heath was obviously oblivious to the thought that someone else could hear him, since he could not hear himself. I also remember a story or 2 of that new go-kart squaring up and running the front end up onto one of the pines they had planted a few year prior. The simple pleasures of living the small-town life as a boy in the country must have made for a very blessed and memorable childhood.

Heath began playing baseball and football as a pretty young kid. The word on the street was he could absolutely fly. I would have loved to watch him play growing up. I have no doubt that quiet, little boy loved to compete to the very end, just like the grown man does that I live with today. He loved everything about practicing and playing ball. He was a born winner, and he was taught to work hard for what you want. Rather than whining when he did not make an all-star team he probably deserved to make, he worked harder in the off season. Today, there are a lot of kids that would greatly benefit from adopting that philosophy.

Heath watched ESPN as a 7-year-old kid, rather than Looney Tunes or Tom & Jerry like most other little boys. He watched football with his daddy and got mad if his mom needed yard work done during a big game on Saturday afternoon. You could say he was a sports guru from the very beginning. He collected the cards. He read the sports magazines. He watched all the different games on TV - and he still loves to do it.

When Heath started school, he and his friends started together at a smaller school that only went through the 8th grade. It was a great place to be and he loved being there. When he was in the 3rd or 4th grade, however, he decided, along with his parents, that moving to the city school would be the only opportunity for him to play baseball and football because it was not offered in the school they started attending. It was a difficult decision they had to make. It was hard to leave many of his good friends behind, but it was a good opportunity for the future.

It was in this new school where his 7th grade science teacher told stories that made Heath think. His teacher had a family that looked a little differently than most of the others he knew. He lived on a farm, complete with milk cows and chickens. They had an orchard, made cheese together and put-up food for the family. His wife supported him from home as she began schooling their children, even though he worked in the public school system. He was a light in the darkness for Heath.

One day Heath was invited to go to the church where his 7th grade science teacher was the pastor. A buddy that lived close by also attended the church, so his mom helped Heath get there, since his parents were working. A strange and peculiar set of events that led him to this church, turned out to be a huge steppingstone in his spiritual life. It was in this church, at a youth retreat, that God called Heath out to be a true follower and disciple of Jesus Christ.

The youth pastor at the church took Heath under his wing. Heath plugged into the youth group and began to grow. He began to see the different paths that some of his friends were taking, but he tried to cling to the truths he was hearing about on Sundays and Wednesdays at church. There were several older men of the church that also invested in Heath's life and the church itself was an opportunity to see families living out their lives the way God intended from the beginning.

Are there people in church that make mistakes? Of course. Do godly people get distracted and veer off the straight and narrow? Absolutely. Are there hypocritical people that sit in the pews on Sunday? We all know the answer is yes. But Heath could see the Lord at work. He did not allow himself to get caught up in the hypocrisy, but rather plugged in to what God was doing.

I can remember Heath telling me that he heard the song, *I Have Decided to Follow Jesus* one night and it was as if his heart was responding to the words of the song. *Though none go with me, I still will follow…no turning back, no turning back.* His desire was to follow the Lord. And from that point on, that was his goal. He wanted to follow Jesus…with his whole heart…for his whole life…whatever that meant…wherever God would lead. Has he made mistakes? Sure. But in no prideful way, the pattern of his life has been one of obedience.

Like any good parent would do, Heath's mom taught her boys how to take care of things that needed doing around the house and in the yard. In the summertime when the boys were home from school, she would leave a list of chores that needed doing before she returned home in the evening. These chores were never overbearing or strenuous, but rather things like folding laundry, sweeping and vacuuming the floors, dusting the furniture or perhaps mowing the lawn. Both of the boys were equally capable of doing all the chores she left them to do and most days they would divide them evenly.

It only took a few days of doing the things on the list, however, to figure out the amount of time they needed to devote to the cleaning. It was soon after this realization that they would choose to play in the yard, swim for a while or watch something on TV in the morning and wait until mid-afternoon to put any effort into the chores they were asked to complete. According to most parents, this is probably normal for the kids that live under their roof as well. Sadly, however, many kids never grow out of this and become procrastinating adults.

As you can probably imagine with two very competitive siblings, everything was a competition, even the chores. It was long into his adult life when Heath confessed to his parents that many days while they were gone to work, the completion of the chore list they left on the counter hinged on who won a game of pool. The kid that was shooting better on that particular day had a whole lot less "work" than the one who struggled. Thankfully, Heath and his brother laid down those pool sticks and both of them work hard to provide for their families today.

It seemed from the outside looking in that Heath was always so independent. He never appeared to need anyone. His parents helped direct him, but he grew and matured much more quickly than many other young men his age. Everyone could see his quiet strength and the leader that he would become. He was one of the older boys that young mothers wanted their little boys to look up to and to follow.

I was intrigued by his personality even from meeting him for the first time. His mom has told me on multiple occasions that God was going to use Heath in big ways. He was a special kind of leader. Obviously, she could not see the future and did not know how things would unfold in his life, but I believe she was right. Truthfully, the events I will share with you in this book very well may be the beginning of God's ultimate plan for Heath, and I am beyond blessed to be a part of it.

Chapter 4
Two Worlds Collide

Two are better than one, because they have
a good reward for their labor.
For if they fall, one will lift up his companion.
But woe to him who is alone when he falls,
for he has no one to help him up.
Ecclesiastes 4:9-10

It is highly debated how long we spend on average at an intersection waiting at traffic lights for a red light to turn green. You may be the type to sit and enjoy the calm and relaxation of the red-light moments. Or maybe you feel rushed and panicked because time is not on your side and the red light is wasting precious minutes of your day. Or perhaps you see the red light as a quick opportunity to gather the random trash that has collected in the floorboard and the cup holders or possibly, you seize the chance to fill out a check to pay the water bill. Today I would consider myself much in line with the multi-tasker - making good use of the down time at the red light. This, however, has not necessarily been the *me* of the past.

There was one specific red light that redirected the course of my life forever. I wish so badly I could remember the exact date, but I guess that small detail is actually irrelevant. One afternoon as I was leaving the cell phone store, where I worked part-time, I was stopped at a red light. My car had no air conditioning, so I had the windows rolled down with my left foot propped up on the door, feeling the wind between my toes. I had plenty of time to get to softball practice, which was just around the corner, so I was actually enjoying the songs on the radio, and I feel certain I was singing along.

Even being the very unobservant person that I am, those few moments being stopped at that specific red light will be burned in my memory forever. I can remember it like it was yesterday even though it was actually about 17 years ago. As my little, grey Camry came to a complete stop, I was instantly aware of the small, baby blue Mitsubishi Galant that was stopped at the same traffic light coming from the opposite direction. The butterflies suddenly came out of nowhere and swarmed around my naive, 20-year-old heart. I had in no way prepared myself for this moment and in the blink of an eye, I was captivated.

He was wearing a black baseball hat with a gold "O" in the center of it. All 4 of his windows were rolled down and he casually made eye contact with me. I was a nervous wreck. My heart was pounding out of my chest, and it was suddenly difficult to swallow, but obviously by his calm and collected demeanor, he was not as captured by this event in history as I was. So, as I tried to maintain my composure and grasped for ideas of how to handle myself for those 90 seconds at the traffic light, I decide that when the light turned green, I would give him a quick glance with a halfway smile and drive straight to ball practice pretending as though the interaction never happened. Were my feelings childish? Perhaps. Ok – YESSS! Do I wish I could re-do the day at the red light? Maybe. But the collision happened that day, perfect or not, and it was the beginning of our lives together. So, no…I would never change it.

Shortly after seeing each other at the red light that day we went separately to a Truth 101 event at the college. It was an event hosted by a local church for college students. A week or 2 later, we began sending emails. Cell phones were not even a thing at the time. If you will think back, you might remember a time when a spiral cord tied you to the wall if you needed to talk on the phone.

It was for this reason, I lived to see a number one on the blue envelope in the top right-hand corner of the computer screen. *I had mail!* And there was only ONE person that sent me mail. It was such a beautiful time. Rather than the "instant gratification" world we live in today, there was a sweet excitement in the anticipation of a phone call and real joy in reading someone's thoughts in an email. Nothing was watered down by simply sharing what others think every day or putting your thoughts out for everyone in the world to read.

There was something intimate that 2 people could share by knowing what another person felt about a certain situation. Even better than that is knowing how they felt about you. Today there is a disconnect in our ability to share our feelings for fear, at least for me, that what is meant to be shared between one heart and another will be copied and pasted for the whole world to weigh in on in a matter of minutes. As a culture we no longer live in the moment, but rather we live to be perceived as having the perfect life. The intimate joys of family are now broadcast for all to see and judge. And all too often our worth is determined by the number of likes and shares our memories have rather than what the One who uniquely created us thinks. Rather than being where our feet are, our minds are constantly pulling us to see what others think of us. We look for positive affirmation from other people, needing to know if they perceive us as being "good enough."

Thankfully, this was not yet reality when our lives together began. We learned a lot about each other through sending those emails back and forth. I shared the fun, exciting details of a most often boring day in paragraph form with him. I asked penetrating questions hoping he might share his deepest feelings with me. He typically responded with very few words, but in a sentence or two he told me he had been thinking of me. It was blissful romance at its finest!!

I can vividly remember one of my professors at the junior college warning me "not to let that cute young man get away from me." She said we were perfect for each other, and she was right. Therefore, my already super-busy life quickly got busier. This handsome guy was often waiting for me as I was finishing up calling the rec league softball games in the evenings. Shortly, I found myself with a 6am running partner at the Nature Trail that circled around the junior college we both attended. There were only a few classes he skipped to play ping-pong in the Student Center with me. I had many more wins than losses, but to his credit, he was not a quitter and I think he enjoyed the challenge.

The local Mexican restaurant learned our favorite foods from the a la carte and they knew we would be drinking water with lemon. In time, I was invited to join his family and him for the Iron Bowl one Saturday afternoon. Sadly, I admit that I slept through a good portion of the game, in front of his dad that I barely knew, but I did wake up in time to help the good team finish out with a win. My car door was always opened for me when we went somewhere together. My daddy even let him drive my car if we needed to take it to town for some reason. I guess I should have known then, he was the man for me.

A gentleman was an understatement. He was 11 months younger than me, but he seemed years older. He had a quiet confidence about him that I was drawn to. He was respectful of my parents' wishes and helped me to see their heart, even when I wanted to be mad about something they did or said. I can remember my outlook changing as I considered taking a spouse, from "maybe he will do" to "there are still guys like this out there?" I had found myself at the point of settling for someone who would "just do." The red light that day gave me a chance for a new perspective. A new life. A new vision. A life that would prove to be the greatest blessing I could have ever imagined.

My parents were obviously in favor of Heath pursuing me, especially since he was the perfect guy. It appeared to them as though he had no flaws anywhere and my father looked for flaws with a fine-toothed comb. I reminisce to that time in our lives together and remember "my" dad wanting to be sure *I* did not "mess it up." Daddy recognized Heath was a man who could lead me spiritually and who could curb my very strong and stubborn personality. Even though I did not know it at the time, my heart longed to be led. It was just going to need a strong man to do it.

Being such an impatient person, there were days before Heath that I felt as if I was out in a wide-open sea of choices. I had no specific direction for my life. I was just as a fish floundering around aimlessly with no real direction in sight. Once I realized Heath was the man I needed to make me whole, my lack of patience intensified quickly. I can remember my mom encouraging me. She would say almost daily, "just walk in the light God gives you." She would remind me that it was okay if I did not know what would happen next week or next month or next year. Truthfully, if I did know, there was a great probability that I would mess it up. She was right, but I was head strong. I felt like I needed the plan. But the Lord made me wait. Looking back, the waiting was for my own good.

Heath never let me push him to expedite the process of

getting married. I was a very "ready to do something" person and I am certain he was quite annoyed at times. He was working on getting things ready behind the scenes; I just did not know it. Neither one of us were high-maintenance people who needed expensive things, so he figured out what he needed to make financially to pay all of our bills without any of my income. Once he had a realistic plan to pay for our basic needs, he found a job at a cabinet shop making just more than he needed to put his plan into action.

The job at the cabinet shop proved to be a tremendous blessing. Heath learned he had a love for wood-working and he also acquired numerous skills that would save us time and money in the near future. I already knew Heath was not afraid of hard work, but in this job, his hard work produced beautiful things. He built kitchen cabinets, bathroom vanities and closet shelving for high-dollar homes. The business he worked for took on several hotels while he was there, outfitting the lobby and entryway with crown molding, hand railing and wainscoting. They built and installed the cabinets and did much of the woodwork and trim as well. It was a huge learning experience for Heath, and he found that he really enjoyed working with wood and he was really good at it.

At some point Heath talked to my dad about us getting married. I had no idea when this took place. He was really good at being mysterious. He told me one time that he carried my engagement ring around for a couple of months in the side pouch of his golf bag that was always in the trunk of his car and I never knew it. We did not know exactly what life would look like, but we both knew we wanted the other one in it. Even before we were engaged, Heath made me feel complete. We were most assuredly better together.

Chapter 5
Making It Legal

Therefore, a man shall leave his father and mother and
be joined to his wife, and they shall become one flesh.
Genesis 2:24

Unfortunately, I have never been overly concerned by my outward appearance. Make-up and jewelry to me in my teen years and early twenties was just for Sunday mornings or possibly a special date night. It may have been that I was just a little lazy and preferred the extra 15 minutes of sleep in the mornings. Perhaps, I just did not care enough about what others thought to take the time to spruce myself up. Either way, my mom frequently encouraged me to put on some pressed powder and a little mascara and to wear something other than faded Nike shorts with an old, stained practice jersey when we went to town.

My sister was quite the opposite. She could rock the gym shorts and t-shirt with me, and she would if we were running together after school or if we were going somewhere after ball practice, but she could also dress with a little more style than I could. At school each day she was always in jeans and a cute shirt or if we went out of town for something she would get fixed up. She wore far more make-up than I did, even on the days I tried. She even washed, dried and fixed her hair - like every day. I always wanted to be cute like she was.

It became a tradition shortly after our move from Mobile to Andalusia that in lieu of birthday presents for each other, my mom, my sister and I would take a day trip together to celebrate. It worked out beautifully because mom was born in February, I celebrated in June and my sister was an October baby. This provided the opportunity at least three times a year for just the three of us to go out for lunch, do a little shopping and just spend some much-needed time together. We all looked forward to the outing. It was nice to slow down for a day, find fun deals at out-of-town thrift stores, eat somewhere other than fast-food and sing, laugh and chat with each other.

On June 10, 2006, we left early on a Saturday morning for Destin, FL. This day was just like many other previous trips we had taken together. It was my birthday "day." My mom and my sister were both dressed cute, but comfortably for the day. They got up early to run the flat iron over their hair. They did their make-up before we left home and they wore some cute earrings and sandals on our little outing. And - then there was me. I was sporting my freshly wrinkled t-shirt straight out of the dryer, my typical athletic shorts, and cheap flip-flops. My hair in a messy ponytail and I was not wearing a stitch of blush or mascara. But we were off to spend the day together and we were all equally excited about it.

We looked forward to the $1 sale on Old Navy flip flops and we often bought a couple of different colors apiece, so this was our first stop of the day. We began to shop, and I found myself in my own little world, browsing through the clearance racks in the very back of the store. I was holding a couple of items in my hand that I had considered trying on. As I turned around to find my mom, hoping to get her opinion of what I had picked out, I was shocked to see Heath walking down the center isle of the store towards me. He was calm and collected and he was holding a dozen roses in his hand. I absolutely love surprises and he certainly had not given me any clues that he would be in Destin that day. I can remember the giddy feeling that took over my heart the moment I saw him, and I hoped so badly that he was staying with us the rest of the day.

His premeditated plan was beginning to unfold as he informed me that I would be leaving with him because he had a surprise. What!?! I love surprises, but just him being there was a surprise. I can remember thinking to myself, *"Can this birthday get any better?"* I felt a little guilty for leaving my mom and my sister until I realized they were in on the plan. I quickly realized why Mom had pushed a little harder than normal for me to change clothes before we left home, and I regretted not taking her advice. Heath acted like he did not care, but I should have tried a little harder getting ready that morning.

His plan was a picnic on the beach. He had thought of everything. He had an old, cozy quilt for us to sit on, my favorite sub with no mayonnaise from Subway, and a football, a frisbee, and extra bottles of water. He also had packed me a little toiletries bag, complete with deodorant, a brush and a razor. He probably knew I would need them. There was also a bathing suit, and a change of clothes, which I assume my mom or his mom helped him get together. My dad was not big on dates, but since my mom knew, I assumed Dad was okay with our little outing. I was as nervous, yet excited as I could be about my birthday date.

Heath and I had the best time on the beach. Because my mom's older brother taught me to throw a frisbee when I was about 8 years old, I thoroughly enjoyed it. He had taught me all kinds of fun tricks to do while catching the frisbee - behind the back, between the legs in stride and my favorite, between the legs with a half turn while in the air. Heath and I loved to goof off. We loved to compete. We loved just being together. We hung out on the beach, competed with frisbee tricks and threw the football for hours. We also enjoyed our picnic of sub sandwiches. I felt special simply because Heath knew me well enough to know what I would order.

I have never been a huge fan of swimming in the saltwater of the Gulf of Mexico, but I do love to walk down the beach. My mom has always loved looking for sand dollars, so I guess I learned to love it from her. On my birthday beach date, Heath and I walked down the beach in the edge of the water. I love feeling the slightly firmer sand beneath my feet that has been packed down by the waves that collapse continuously onto the shore.

I talked non-stop every step down the beach about every thought that entered my mind. He listened and would occasionally respond with a word or two, so I would know he was still listening. I savored our time on the beach together. I felt completely loved and cared for. I was the most important thing in the world to him in those moments. I was aware, however, that our time together would be coming to an end because the sun would be quickly approaching the horizon. After some piece down the beach, we turned our backs to sun and began making our way back towards the old quilt that was still resting on the sand holding all of our stuff.

My heart was so full and my love tank was overflowing from this thoughtful, surprising gesture from the one who made me tick. I felt certain that this was obvious to him of course, since I had showered him with numerous words and thoughts on our relaxing stroll down the beach and back. I felt sure that he desperately wanted to hear everything, great or small, that I had ever felt, for that is how I felt about him. Therefore, I pelted him with my thoughts for the entirety of our walk. Thinking back, I can see why the bible says to be quick to listen and slow to speak. That night his ears were probably pleading for a break and longing for silence, but I am a work in progress, and he made it through the lovely evening.

Just before we arrived back to our old quilt on the beach, I guess I took a short breath and glanced back at the sun as it was beginning to set. When I turned back around, thinking of something else to blab about, Heath was on one knee. He had a small, hand-made, wooden ring box he built for me at the cabinet shop he was working in. It was holding a beautiful 3/4 carat solitaire with a solid, gold band. It was perfect. Completely unexpected. A breathtaking moment I will not soon forget. I am certain the tears quickly began to flow, and I can remember it being hard to even speak the word, "Yes," even though every fiber of my being wanted to scream it at the top of my lungs. It is so strange how a few minutes prior to this, there were a plethora of words flowing freely from my heart, but in this moment, I was speechless.

Being with Heath made everything in life right for me. Even the hard moments. The times I was uncertain or confused. Even the times of discomfort. He was always my rock solid, even from the beginning. I felt complete when I was with him and I wanted him to feel the same completeness when he was with me. He never said that he did, but he did ask me to marry him, so I figure that was close enough.

I would not be truthful if I were to say that Heath and I discussed all of the ways that we would be better suited for the kingdom of God if we were to get married. We never discussed all the aspects of theology that some Christians do before marriage. I can recall a conversation or 2 regarding children and my desire was to have none. We did discuss and ultimately decided, at the request of my dad, that we would *live* on Heath's salary alone and that everything I made would either be saved, used for a vacation, or to pay down on something, but we would never *depend* on my income to pay the bills. Other than that, we knew that God brought us together, so with our parent's approval, we decided to dive in and see where the Lord would lead us.

We immediately began thinking about a December wedding. He was also in school, so it would give us 6 months or so to plan. He would have a break from classes for the holiday and it would give us time to find a place to live. It seemed like the wisest choice to make. However, I find it hard to sit still for any length of time, so I quickly got to work searching for a place to live. We were only a couple of weeks into the wedding planning when we found a place to rent within our budget. Heath had a full-time job making enough money to pay all of our bills with his paycheck alone. With that being said, we decided September would work perfectly for us.

And so it was that our 2-month and 2-week long engagement came to a close on September 2, 2006. We were just 2 kids madly in love with each other, but totally willing to work hard for what we wanted, which was life together. We were completely confident that we were better together than we were apart. We knew it was not going to be easy and we never anticipated a "rosy" life together. There was plenty of discouragement for us from people who wanted us to live the perfect American Dream, but we did not need perfection. We just needed each other.

Heath was only 21 years old, and I was the ripe old age of 22 when we made our vows to each other. Of course, there were numerous people who questioned our decision not to wait awhile longer – wait until we finished school…wait to save some more money…wait to grow up a little more…wait until we could buy a nice place to live…wait and enjoy life a little first. But, with the Lord's blessing, we knew we wanted to build a life together. And, I would like to think, we are currently living it – the American dream. Even though it has taken more work on our part than most people are willing to put forth and more sacrifices in the short term than many people are willing to make in hopes of reaping the long-term rewards, the Lord has been so good to us.

I can honestly say I have never regretted starting our lives together so early in life. The Lord has been so faithful to lead our family even from the earliest stages of our lives together. He has provided all of our "needs," along with some of our "wants" as well. We have never done without.

It was not our plan when we said "I do" to have 6 children in the span of 11 years. It was also not a part of our plan for me to quit my job to stay home and raise our children, but the Lord has allowed us to grow through the struggles of discomfort. He has allowed us to reap the benefits of trusting in Him. Life together has had specific challenges that we never saw coming, but even in those times, I have always been led. Heath looks to the Lord for his strength and therefore, he can lead me. He is without a doubt my strong and steady, small-town handsome man, who loves me even when I do not deserve it.

Chapter 6
The Calm before the Storm

Come now, you who say, "Today or tomorrow we will go to such and such a city, spend a year there, buy and sell, and make a profit;" whereas you do not know what will happen tomorrow. For what is your life? It is even a vapor that appears for a little time and then vanishes away.
James 4:13-14

I will skip quickly through the next 12 – 13 years of our married lives together and I will pick back up on a cool November afternoon in 2018. Heath came home from work and the kids were doing feet-off-the-floor. Feet-off-the-floor is a 45-minute rest period I created where all the kid's feet must stay off the ground and they cannot use their voices at all. They are permitted to read a book, draw or color in their bed (the older kids only) or take a short nap. After a long, productive school day, this allowed me to take a few minutes to get supper in the works and to take a quick breather before Heath got home from work.

Heath was a lineman for the local power company. Most days he worked hard and he appreciated me creating a time to unwind a bit before he got home as much or more than I enjoyed taking the quick break from answering questions and refilling sippy cups. I was less inclined to bombard him with *all* the details of the day, so he was able to relax for a few minutes after a long day at work. It was a win-win for everyone.

Many days I would sit in the recliner in the living room with my Bible, my journal and a cup of coffee. I tried to time feet-off-the-floor so that it would coincide with the baby's nap time. As a mom, I have often found it difficult to spend any quality time in prayer or in the Word. Many times, I found myself frustrated because I tried to make the time, but a nursing baby or a hard night with no sleep made it quite difficult. This time in the afternoon felt like a refuge if I was able to make all the stars align perfectly, so that I was able to enjoy those few minutes alone. I would pray or start supper or plan my grocery list or even just sit and think while I sipped on an afternoon cup of coffee. This particular day, all the details had come together perfectly and there I was nestled in the corner of the living room by the fireplace in the recliner when Heath quietly opened the door and stepped into the entryway.

He made a cup of coffee and joined me in the living room. With seemingly no thought at all, he casually mentioned a piece of property that he had always loved and wondered who owned it. "Do you ever think about selling our house," he calmly asked me. *What?* I thought. *Well, actually I have thought about it many times, but this is our forever home…right!?! We had a housewarming and everything! This is a huge house that the Lord has blessed us with. For almost six months, we lived in a 12x24 schoolroom you built for me while we remodeled the whole inside of this house. We worked so hard. It has funky angles that I love and the cabinets you built for me are exactly what I have always longed to have. Sure, there are more things we need to do, but it has come so far. I love this house and I am completely comfortable here and now you are asking me if I want to leave!?!* My reply however was much different than my thoughts. "Well," I calmly replied while inwardly screaming, "Let's see if we can figure out who owns the land."

Through asking around at work and a couple of nifty apps he found on his phone, Heath located the property owner and inquired about buying the piece of land that was not even for sale. You guessed it…we bought it. The grass on this piece of land we purchased was head high in most places. It had dead limbs cluttering much of the ground and the entire property was covered with poison oak. But we have always enjoyed "projects," so we made the plan to tackle it.

Since we did not have a tractor, my first thought after seeing the land for the first time was "elbow grease" – lots of elbow grease. This property would need a ton of hard work to ever come close to making what was once a beautiful piece of real estate even slightly appealing again. At one time the acreage was the resting place of a 4,000 square foot home, which contained separate living quarters on two different levels. Many years ago, the home burned to the ground leaving nothing but the slab of concrete on the lowest level and a portion of the retaining wall which once created the basement portion of the home. What once was a well-groomed and perfectly manicured home was now nothing but a pile of rubble and a huge undertaking in the making. But, if this was where the Lord was leading Heath, I was willing to follow him there.

Even though our budget allowed us to purchase the property and continue saving as we had been previously, we were still unsure how or why this land was laid so heavily on Heath's heart and furthermore, how in the world we bought almost 6 acres in a prime location for our area that was not even for sale. It was mind-boggling. Thinking back, we were so very certain that it was what the Lord was leading us to do and He worked out detail after detail to begin unfolding His plan right in front of our very eyes.

We prayed for months, and we ask the Lord to give us wisdom. Many times, we knelt together and asked to Lord to confirm in us His will for our family. We knew the looks and questions we would get if we proceeded to sell our house with 4 bedrooms, 2 baths and 11 acres of secluded land. We had spent a solid year working to create a safe, peaceful, homey refuge away from the craziness of the fallen world we live in. Our oasis was even complete with a huge tree house that Heath built for the kids. It was ah-mazing. He added a 12-foot rock wall to one side, a 16-foot rope swing to the other, monkey bars and a turquoise chandelier hanging in the living space. The ladder into the tree house had a thick, off-white rope handrail and each step was beveled at the top to make it pretty to look at and easier to walk up and down. The kids spent hours a day climbing, pretending and enjoying the work and creativity of their daddy's hands. And he enjoyed every minute of building it.

It seemed the more we thought and the more we talked, the more we felt led that this house we loved was not where we would grow old together. We had no idea what selling a house would mean, nor did we even know where to start, but we dove in headfirst trying to take steps to put our house on the market. We prayed daily that the Lord would warn us if we were making a mistake. The questions came and numerous people expressed their own opinions of what we were about to do, but we were confident that we were being led to sell it. The times of deepest doubt were always met with affirmation that could only come from the Lord himself. He confirmed in us that we were in His will.

The house was posted on a website for selling homes and we sold it in less than 40 days from the day we posted it. Obviously, Heath and I neither one knew anything at all about the logistics of selling a home, so both of us were somewhat nervous. We wanted to be certain that we did everything correctly at closing. But just like God does, He practically provided us with a real estate agent through the people that purchased our house. She may never even know it, but she was a tremendous blessing to us. The Lord used her in one of the most stressful times of our marriage. She took a tremendous amount of stress off of both of us and we are grateful to her even to this day for taking us under her wing.

So, during this crazy endeavor, 10 days before we closed on the sale of our house, we had nothing to call home except a grown up, messy piece of land. You hear people say, the Lord works in mysterious ways, and He certainly did for us. The week we closed on the house, a buddy Heath worked with decided to sell his 31-foot RV with double slide outs. You can probably guess where this is going. Yep. We bought it. I know…and bought it to LIVE in. Everyone said we were crazy, and honestly, they were right. But Heath went to work like a madman. I have never seen someone with such raw talent.

He formulated the plan and quickly put it into action. Along with a lot of strength from my brother and the know-how of a very dear friend and mentor, Heath built a large pole barn on the piece of land we had purchased. It was perfect. The camper was backed under the barn he built on a Wednesday. We slept there for the first time that night before even having it leveled. He laid down the water lines and a friend helped him get the power to it the next day and we were set.

A long 2 days later, we began the final walk-through of what we thought was the home we would grow old together in. It was a bit emotional, for me especially, but we were trying to move forward and be obedient to the Lord the best way we knew how. We were so confident in the Lord's calling on our lives, that we have not looked back since that day.

Camper life is not for the faint of heart, especially if your husband is 6′ 3″ and the shower head doesn't even reach your head or if you enjoy a plush, comfy mattress when you lie down after a long, hard day, but it is totally doable. If you ever choose to give this lifestyle a valiant effort, I would recommend a minimum of 2 crock pots, something to create some resemblance of a porch and as thick of a mattress topper as you can find. It will certainly help you find the difference in what you "need" and what you "want." Quickly, we found that a way to wash clothes for 8 people was a need, so Heath built a utility room on the back side of the pole barn. It had everything I needed – a washer and dryer, a stand-up freezer and a place to house extras that I could not fit in the camper. He even sealed it up well for me. I will gladly choose NO critters in my laundry room over A/C in the dead of summer.

Our family was packed like sardines in that little camper, but it was the sweetest and most intimate time together. We lived on little for a little while, but we all have a new appreciation for the simple things in life as a result of our camping adventure. Of course, the tight-nit-ness of our new situation caused us to work quickly putting our newly created plan into motion. Well, it actually was not a "new" plan because we have dreamed for years of how we might become debt-free.

Heath's goal had always been to be debt-free by the time he was 50 years old and I made it my mission to help him achieve that plan. Certainly, there have been sacrifices, but we wanted to live like no one else, so one day we can live like no one else – in freedom. To most people, financial freedom is not even considered, but I believe it is a common desire we both wanted badly enough to put our heads together and create a plan. It was somewhat drastic in the beginning, but it felt so good to see the Lord begin to bless our efforts as we sought His face.

The dream we shared was to build a shop with living quarters. This would allow Heath to have the space he needed to do the woodworking he would need to do, while allowing us to live in a 2 bedroom, 2 bath house with a kitchen and living area. Our plan was to continue to save money as we lived in what seemed to most to be a "tiny house." We then would build what we hoped would be the home where our children could bring their friends and special-some-ones for us to get to know. We would eventually sit together in white rocking chairs on the front porch, while watching our grandchildren play in the yard or on the porch at our feet. So…the plan began taking shape. I put my ideas on paper for the tiny house – in a notebook, on the back of an envelope or with dry erase marker on the mirror - and Heath made them come to life.

Heath learned as he built, but our little house began taking shape. He continued working his full-time job, while building a place for us to live. I designed the kid's bathroom with 2 potties, 2 showers and 2 make-up areas along with a space that would hold 10 full-size laundry baskets for storage and organized laundry. Heath measured, plumbed and constructed everything to make the practically unique bathroom, and entire house for that matter, all that I ever hoped it could be. Heath also built 2 sets of triple bunk beds, so the kids would each have their own sleeping space. There is certainly a unique preciousness about standing in the doorway of that small bedroom and looking into the eyes of all my children in one little space that just makes my heart full. To me it is perfect. The shop with living quarters took Heath about 6 months to build.

We were able to move in around the end of the September. We still lacked a few things, like baseboards, a few door casings and our porches. It took us a little while to settle in, but we were getting things in place by Christmas. We cut a live Christmas tree for the first time that year. Everything in our lives at that time seemed a bit more "living." People still thought we were crazy for what we had chosen to do, but I saw our home as a direct blessing from the Lord and as another step in the process of achieving the dream we longed to reach together – financial freedom.

I will skip through the holiday season and pick back up here on the evening of January 27, 2021. This was the night before the accident, but it ended as any other normal Wednesday night would for our family. The church we attended did not even assemble for the mid-week service until 7pm. They did, however, provide a meal, so I did not have to feed hungry kiddos when we got home. Heath and I had been serving in the college class ministry at church for almost 10 years. Heath had been teaching through the book of Acts.

In combination with all the other events that happen during a normal work week, a Wednesday night is probably the hardest night of the week for our family. We are tired…like, really tired. A typical drive home from church on Wednesday night means that as we are headed into the driveway, Heath will ask the kids what he is about to say. They know the drill – teeth, pajamas, bed - literally as quickly as humanly possible. They know that if there is a night *not* to test daddy, this is it. He and I both are running on fumes, and we are longing to lie down in the bed of our own.

I guess I am living in a glass house as I give an account of God's provision for me. I have already shared with you a few of the exciting and miraculous details of our living arrangements, so that night, all 6 of our children snuggled down in the same bedroom. They slept on two sets of triple bunk beds that were uniquely positioned on top of each other so that each child would have room to sit up and turn over without hitting the bed above or below them. Almost every night Heath and I make the round from top to bottom and then from bottom to top kissing each one of our little people. They feel safe as we stand in the doorway of their bedroom, with the noise maker humming softly in the background, as Heath prays over them. He will thank the Lord for His protection over our family. He will pray for those who are hurting and in need of healing and he asks the Lord for wisdom as he seeks to lead our family. It is a time we all look forward to each night.

After he finished praying that night, we turned out the lights in the majority of the house. Heath locked the doors, as he always does, and we slowly dragged ourselves off to bed. I usually lie awake for hours trying to fall asleep, even though my body is exhausted. Heath, on the other hand, is asleep within 45 seconds of his head resting on the pillow. At least my lack of sleep does not keep him awake…*I guess.*

The next morning, I was half-asleep walking around in the half-lit kitchen making a pot of coffee. Life does not begin for me each day until I have had at least two cups of coffee and even then, it is slowly that I begin to gain consciousness. Heath is different. He wakes up in a good mood, ready to take on the day. He has the same routine every morning. He does everything in the same order, the same way, every day. Maybe that is the reason I lose my phone on a daily basis, but he has only forgotten his wallet or his phone twice in the entirety of our marriage.

I love to watch him. He could get ready for work every day blindfolded because he has perfected the routine. It is quite humorous, however, to move something on the dresser from one side to the other. It throws off his morning rhythm. He is kind and loving, however, when I feel the need to rearrange things. He never gripes or complains when I need to change the placement of his phone charger…so that I can change the location of the lamp…in order to add a picture to the dresser…so that I can decorate the mantle for newest season. He just adapts to the new and adjusts the routine.

This particular morning, he was to be at work at 6am. The

routine had gone as normal and thus continued as he slipped on his work boots in the mudroom. He grabbed his lunchbox and walked out into the chilly air to start his truck. When he came back inside, I met him at the door in my pajamas with his cup of coffee in my hands. I put my arms inside his camel colored Carhartt jacket and asked him to take me with him to work in my best whiny voice. He wrapped me up inside his jacket, prayed over our day and kissed me as he walked out the door about 5:25am. I could see the headlights cutting through the blackness of the yard and I called for him to hurry home to see me. Though I cannot remember exactly what I did after closing the door and locking it behind him, my best guess is that I laid back down in our bed that was still warm, since I had most likely only slept a couple of hours during the night. I would typically use his pillow instead of mine just because it smelled like him and I wanted him to be close to me.

My alarm went off a short while later. I got up, made more coffee and got the kids up and going. We made quick use of our school day, making sure that we tackled math and grammar, but we had an early afternoon appointment to visit with my grandmother who lived in town. She was in need of some kids with strong backs to take the garbage to the dumpster and to do a few other seemingly small tasks.

While the kids were helping her, I made myself busy reorganizing her guest bedroom closet. She was helping me bag up items to give to the less fortunate and I was labeling the drawers for the numerous purses in a wide array of shades and sizes that she was not yet willing to part with. I was deep in conversation with her, attempting to persuade her that more than 30 purses just was not necessary, but I was interrupted by my phone ringing. I could hear the sound, but I could not find it buried beneath all of the clutter we had created on the bed. When I finally answered the phone, I began walking to her front porch so that I could hear a little better.

The number I had saved was one of Heath's co-workers, so I expected it to be Heath calling from his number. In a very calm, nonchalant way, his buddy asked me if I had heard from Heath. I explained to him that there was a little trouble on one of the switches and Heath told me he would be late getting home from work, but he thought he would finish in time for our daughter's basketball game that evening. His friend said he had heard there was some trouble, but he was in his tree stand in the woods, so it must be nothing. Within 20 seconds of hanging up the phone, my phone rang again. This time it was Heath. I knew the second I heard his voice that something was wrong.

"Hey, Rach," Heath said to me. "I just wanted you to know there has been an accident. I don't really know what happened, but I wanted you to hear it from me and I want you to know I am ok." I asked if he was at the hospital to which he responded, "Not yet, but I am going to be." I told him not to worry and reassured him that I would figure out the details and I would see him soon. The phone call from Heath was heavy, but looking back on my recent call log, the conversation lasted less than sixty seconds. There was no fear in Heath's voice, but my heart could feel the gravity of his situation.

Immediately, I called the co-worker back to ask questions. What could be wrong? How bad could it be? What should I do now? I remember very little of that conversation, but I vividly remember him saying these words: "Rachel, if Heath can speak to you, he is going to be alright."

The Lord used the words Heath's buddy spoke to me in those moments to still my heart and remind me to pray. I began to beseech the Lord to intervene. I had no idea what was going on, but I knew He knew exactly. In my naive mind, the "accident" could have been a car wreck or Heath could have fallen from a pole he was climbing. Maybe a piece of equipment malfunctioned or something of that nature. Regardless of what happened, he needed the omnipotent healing hand of the Creator at that very moment. And so, we prayed.

I gathered all of the kids and asked my grandmother to join us. The kids and I, along with my grandmother who stood proudly with us at the age of 92 years, held hands in a circle. We were standing in the parking lot of her apartment complex calling out to the Lord on behalf of our daddy. Even though, I had no idea what type of "accident" Heath was referring to, I knew I had to get to where he was. We pleaded with the Lord in those moments to intervene on our behalf. We asked the Lord to protect Heath and to give the doctors wisdom as they tried to care for him.

Of course, I did not verbalize this specific prayer while I was still with my children, but I can remember asking the Lord to help me make it to the hospital to see Heath alive. I had no idea what had actually happened, but I could sense in Heath's voice when he said, "I'm ok," he meant in life or in death. He was at peace with losing his life and strangely enough, I had the same peace. I knew that Heath was right with his Creator and that he would simply be in paradise with our heavenly Father before I would be. But even knowing that, I still longed to see his face again. I had no idea what to expect, but I can remember hoping he would be able to touch my skin with his big, strong hands and that he would be conscious enough to know I was there.

As I loaded the kids up in the car, hugged my grandmother good-bye and started out of the apartment complex, I can still feel my heart pounding as I tried to figure out where to go. I called grandparents and siblings, but no one answered the phone. As I continued trying to contact someone to tell me where Heath was going to be, I quickly developed a plan for the kids. I was going to leave the kids at my sister's house and put the oldest ones in charge of the younger. Thankfully though, when I pulled into the driveway, I could see her car. Instant relief. As the kids piled out of the car, tears already streaming from some of their faces, other ones having no clue what was going on, we said our good-byes. My heart was broken leaving them. Honestly, I had no idea when I would be back to get them, but it seemed like the right thing to do, so I left.

Moments after I pulled out of her driveway, Heath's supervisor who was at the scene of the accident, called me back. I inquired which local hospital Heath would be going to and I can remember his response like it was yesterday. He said, "The helicopter will be here in just a few minutes, and I have heard Sacred Heart in Pensacola." As I hung up the phone, my mind was racing. *What? Sacred Heart in Pensacola? Helicopter…meaning Life Flight?? How is this even possible?? I literally JUST talked to him on the phone…*

Eight-Year-Old Fear

By: Ollie Williamson

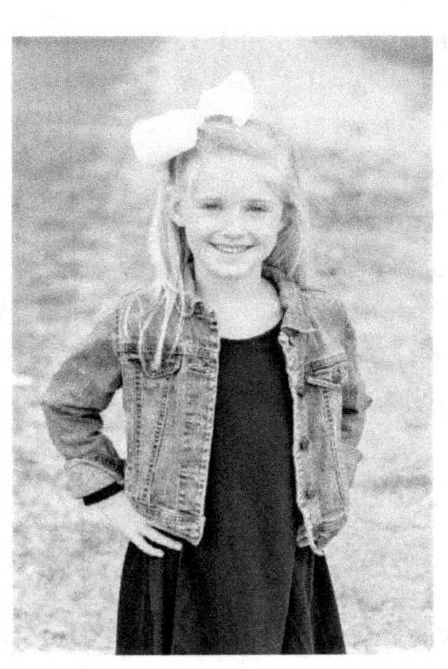

I was 8 years old when daddy had the accident. Mom got us out of the car to pray for Daddy after she heard what happened. I was so scared. I cried in the back seat of the car all the way to Annie's house. I thought Daddy might already be dead.

After mom left, we all held hands in the living room and prayed for daddy. I tried to sit down and play with the toy trains, but all I wanted was to know if Daddy was ok.

Chapter 7
Calmly Scattered

When times are good, be happy;
but when times are bad, consider:
God has made the one as well as the other.
Ecclesiastes 7:14 (NIV)

As I think back to the few moments when I dropped our children off at my sister's house, I feel the guilt all over again. I knew I needed to remain calm and to try and gather my thoughts, but I remember feeling frazzled. I do not think I ever panicked, but I was probably pretty close to it. I had no idea how long I would be gone when I left them that day. I had very little information to share with them. I never wanted to give them a false hope that Heath would survive, nor did I want them to give up hope while he was still with us. I am sure they felt fear from the uncertainty of the situation. I am sure they questioned if they would ever see their daddy again. He was our rock solid. He was the anchor of our home. Everyone that lived under the roof of our house turned to him for comfort, leadership and wisdom. He loved, protected and provided for each one of his children, the same way he had always done for me.

While going through the process of calling his parents and

mine to inform them of what little I knew, I drove mindlessly around in circles trying to remember the way to my house. I desperately needed tears to come, but they would not. Once I got to my house, I began putting things I thought I might need in a bag to take to the hospital.

Suddenly, in the midst of packing, I found myself frozen. Standing in the middle of my bathroom staring out the window, I was in a trance. I needed my mind to think and to process what I should do next, but I was stunned. I guess a form of shock had taken over my body. It felt like it lasted for several minutes.

Out of nowhere, I heard my phone ring and it snapped my mind back into reality. For no particular reason and having no idea what was going on, my brother called my phone. He had not heard the news. I guess my voice told him something was wrong. I explained to him what little I knew and asked him to pray with me. He was calm and reassuring. After our conversation, he went to work ironing out details for a place he knew I would need to stay later that night.

Heath's mom picked me up at my house. I am so thankful she was in town and close by so that I did not have to make a 2+ hour drive alone. We discussed the surface possibilities of what might have happened, but neither one of us wanted to verbalize the possibility of losing the one we loved. I think we both needed someone to hold us, giving us the opportunity to unleash all of the emotions that were beginning to build up after learning about the situation and the anticipation of what was to come. But because the arms were not there, the strength to hold it together continued.

Heath's daddy was on the road driving a truck when I called to tell him the news of the accident. He is a living, breathing roadmap, so he created a place on our way for us to meet him. We met him at a truck-stop just off the interstate as we headed south. I can remember watching him back that 18-wheeler into the parking spot, leaving the keys in the truck, grabbing his bag and walking towards me. I anticipated being able to fall apart in his arms as he hugged me in the middle of that truck stop parking lot, but as soon as his arms were around me, I was aware it was Heath I needed. I instantly understood it was not just "an" embrace I longed for, but rather it was for the arms of the only man who was the gatekeeper and protector of my heart.

As we continued on from there, the sun was setting on the horizon. Our destination was no longer Pensacola, but rather the Emergency Room at University Hospital in Mobile, AL. We had no idea where to go or what to ask, but led by his flashers, Heath's dad hit 110mph on the interstate as we headed towards the hospital. It was completely dark once we arrived. I walked under the large, red, illuminated sign that read *Emergency Room*. I told the lady at the front desk who I was. I could tell by the buzz behind the desk, that everyone was aware of the situation and that it was not something they saw every day.

I was taken to a small holding room inside the emergency room waiting area. The head paramedic that night was a very kind and gentle man. I believe he could sense the anxiety of my heart and he did his best to speak calming words to me. He had previously worked for a large power company in Alabama, which primarily deals with transmission power lines. Transmission lines, for those of you who do not already know, are the larger power lines that feed the substations for smaller distribution companies. The smaller lines are used to light up our homes and businesses. I only knew the difference because Heath also worked on those *larger transmission lines* and I knew the danger associated with such work.

This kind man in the waiting room tried to encourage me with these words and they will be burned in my memory forever. He said to me, "Sweetheart, you should be so thankful your husband wasn't working on transmission lines or he would not still be here." I could see the genuine expression on his face, but he had no idea what he had just told me. Those were the words that told me what *actually* happened. Electrocution. Heath had been electrocuted.

After coming to fully understand the gravity of the situation, my cluttered mind began to process – transmission lines?? Quickly, I understood the Lord's grace in allowing me to be in the dark while I left my children crying and while I made the drive to the hospital. His timing was perfect in allowing this sweet man to inform me of what really took place in Heath's bucket truck a few hours prior, so I only had a few moments to think about it before I saw Heath face to face.

My mind immediately began to pray, "Father, prepare my heart. Do not allow my face to show anything that is not in my heart. I do not care what he looks like or what I am about to see, but please guard my expressions and please Lord, help him know that I am here." Heath had talked to the kids in the past about the dangers of electricity. I knew what "should" happen if someone was exposed to the electrical voltage – especially the amount of voltage that he worked with - and I did not know how to prepare myself mentally.

I knew that a blue electrical arc should blind a person, so I wondered if he would be able to see me, if he was even still conscious. I prepared myself for his eyes to be black and his skin to be charred. I did not know until days later that electrical burns are different from most other types of burns. They begin on the inside and work towards the outside. I thought of all the possibilities you might consider. I was fully prepared for this to be the end for Heath. Surely his organs were fried.

I have always called him Superman. He can literally do anything, but he is mortal. Surely this would be the end of our lives together. With every breath I felt myself leaning on the Lord for help and pleading with the Lord for a miracle, yet preparing my heart for the worst – earthly separation from the one my heart loved.

I did not understand why this was part of God's plan. I had no idea how I would survive under what I knew was coming. I called out, minute after minute to the Lord for help. I only waited a few minutes in that small waiting room, but it seemed like an eternity. Heath had a close friend who was working with him in the bucket at the time of the accident. His buddy suffered worse burns on his hands and arms than Heath did, so he was taken into surgery first. Shortly after his buddy was taken to the Operating Room, I was called back to see Heath. There were doctors and nurses scurrying around his bedside like ants, trying to formulate a plan.

His eyes were glassy, but seemingly unharmed. It was hard to maintain eye contact with him in those moments, and I did not know why. His skin was rather pale and he was cool to the touch. He had several cords that were used to monitor different things stuck to his chest and hanging from his ear. Even though there were people everywhere asking questions, needing signatures, and busy making a plan, I could still hear the soft, unnatural rhythm of his heartbeat in the background. His heart was in A-fib. The doctors gave us 18 hours to correct the rhythm of his heart with medicine. If it was unsuccessful, they would try to stop his heart and shock it back into rhythm.

I was so thankful to finally see him and yet my heart would not allow me to accept what I saw as reality. I was guarded. I was prepared for the inevitable. I quickly put boundaries around my heart and my emotions to lessen the pain I would feel when he was gone. Rather than looking to the miracle-working, sovereign hand of God that intervened in the bucket truck earlier that day, I allowed all the facts and figures to seep into my mind and heart. Those things caused me to question what I believed. The things I was told and the feelings that I felt, distracted me.

As I looked around, taking in every detail of our last moments together, I could feel the peace in Heath's spirit. He was not afraid and even in that hospital bed, he was my strength. His right hand and forearm were still slightly convulsing. They were so large; I was afraid they would burst. He had charred, oblong spots on the bottoms of both feet. In addition to the electricity coming in and out the bottoms of both feet, he also had a large hole in the back of his right calf. The work clothes they cut off of him were laying in a pile on the floor beside the gurney where he was lying. He whispered to me, "I don't know what is going to happen, but I want you to know, I love you."

The on-call doctor that night was a plastic surgeon, and she would eventually do the emergency surgery shortly after I met her. She came to his bedside, her shoulders barely reaching the top of the bed, and explained what needed to happen. "Mr. Williamson," she explained. "I do not know if we can save your right hand or not, but we will need to do surgery immediately to even give ourselves a chance." She was genuine, compassionate and ready to act.

I stood beside his bed, with an occasional tear rolling down my face, waiting for them to come and take him to the operating room. I can remember gently running my fingers through his hair and letting him know I would be there waiting when he came out. In my mind, however, this was the last time I would see him alive. As they came to take him to surgery, I walked alongside the bed as far as I could. When they asked me to stop, I gave him what I thought was our last kiss, and let him go. I snapped a quick picture with my phone, so I would never forget the moment.

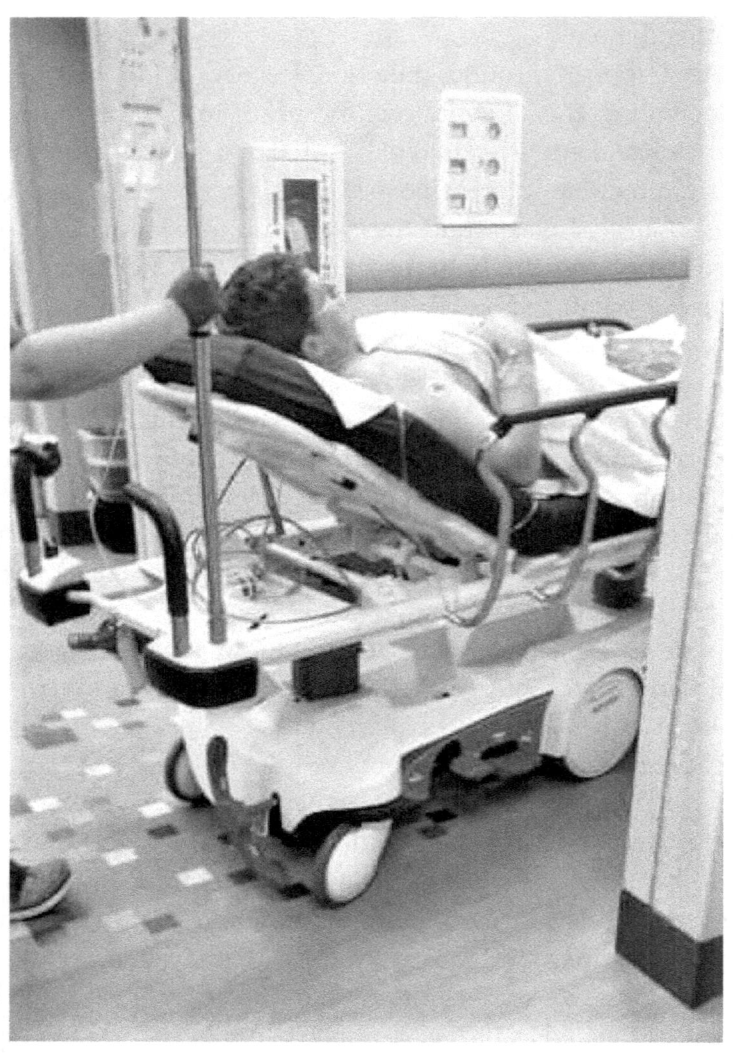

In my mind, this was the last time I would see him alive. I walked alongside the bed as far as I could. When they asked me to stop, I gave him what I thought was our last kiss, and let him go.

I waited that night for hours. Finally, I got a call that he was out of surgery and had been moved to a recovery room. Even though my husband survived the emergency surgery that night, I was not allowed to see him. New rules and regulations had been put in place as a result of tremendous fear that had swept through our country. It just felt wrong. It *was* wrong. I needed him and he needed me.

The hospital also would not allow his parents to see their son who was fighting for his life. It was a shameful thing that added to the emotional struggle in my heart that night. Even though I knew they would not let me go back to see him, I just could not make myself leave the hospital. I wanted to be where Heath was. I could feel my heartbeat pounding away in my head and my body felt so weak, but I knew I would never go to sleep even if I tried. My aunt and uncle, who both still live in Mobile, came by and brought me a sandwich. Thinking back, I do not even remember them being there, but they loved me by meeting a physical need I had that night – food.

Several people came to the hospital to be with Heath's parents and me, some of which I had never met. The kind words people spoke in that waiting room about my husband, had to be genuine. I knew in my heart, they were not merely words, because they knew the same man I knew. Heath was real - day in and day out, and obviously those people knew that about him just like I did. Those words touched my soul and gave me a new sense of pride in the man who was fiercely fighting for his life that night.

We left the hospital to get some rest just before 4am. I was told I could see Heath when the hospital opened the next morning at 8am. I wish I could tell you that I slept during those long, 4 hours in a foreign hotel room, but if I slept at all, it certainly was not much. Heath's daddy dropped me off at the entrance of the hospital at 8am on the dot. He was my human compass and road map in the city where I was born and raised. Even if I had a good sense of direction, which I certainly do not, I was slightly distracted, and I would have never found my way to and from the hospital without him. I made my way up to the 4th floor. It housed the ICU Burn Unit, which is where Heath was taken after surgery. It was required that I dress in a lovely, yellow, tear-away gown that covered my clothing. I also got to adorn my hair with a beautiful blue hair net and of course, I was required to wear a facemask. I felt like these things were silly, just like many of the other new rules in place at the hospital, but it was definitely worth it to be able to see Heath again. The kids sent Heath cards and letters that I taped to the walls of the hospital for him to see.

Not long after arriving that morning, one of the sweet ICU nurses came into our room. She asked Heath in her high-pitched, almost laughing voice, "Mr. Williamson. We have 115,000 volts of electricity in your chart. Uhm…is that a misprint?" He was half-way smiling and said, "No ma'am. It isn't. I know – I shouldn't be here right now." Her eyes were the size of saucers, and she was totally speechless. She did not even respond, but slowly turned around and walked out of the room.

It was that evening when I found myself alone in the hotel room that I was able to google the amount of voltage used to execute someone in the electric chair. I was shocked by the information I received from the simple google search. It felt like my heart would stop as I read statements like…the first, more powerful jolt (between 2,000 and 2,500 volts) of electric current is intended to cause immediate unconsciousness and cardiac arrest…the second jolt of 500-1,500 volts is intended to cause fatal damage to vital organs…a shock above 2,700 volts will kill a person or cause severe injury…and the facts continued. Suddenly, what I knew in my head was becoming reality in my heart. I should be at home…alone…with just my children…planning my husband's funeral.

There are so many details I could give of just the stay in the ICU Burn unit. Most of it consists of numerous doctors and nurses coming in and out, asking questions and formulating a plan for the next few surgeries to clean up everything that was dead in Heath's body. It was vital to get him ready for skin grafts and/or plastic surgery. The medicine was effective in reestablishing Heath's normal heartbeat, but we had so many other issues to contend with. They ranged from an allergic reaction to the bed sheets he was lying on to him not being able to pee after they took the catheter out. It seemed like one thing after another.

Being removed a couple of days from the accident had allowed me to process and gather my thoughts to some degree, but things were happening so quickly, I could not keep up. A very dear friend gifted me a journal, a box of cards and some fun pens with different colored ink. Those were the most precious items anyone could have given me at that time. I needed to get my thoughts and feelings outside of my brain, but if I tried to speak them, I just sounded like a cluttered mess. It was a mess, but writing the words described, even to me, what I was actually feeling.

One of the first entries in my journal was this:

Jan 30, 2021
10:30am

Something worthy to note: Heath woke up suddenly and asked me to find this verse for him. He is back asleep now, so I will write it here.

"But these things are written that you may believe that Jesus is the Christ, the Son of God, and that by believing you may have life in his name." John 20:31 (NIV)

I was reminded even as I wrote those words down onto paper, that the Word of the Lord is very much alive. This scripture was at the very core of who Heath was. Being unsure if he would even survive to the next day, his desire was that all men who heard about his situation would be able to understand that their greatest need was to know Christ personally. It was so gripping as I thought about it personally. I questioned of my own self, what would flow out of my heart if our roles were reversed? What would be in my heart of hearts if I were potentially staring death on this earth in the face?

Jan 30, 2021
11:35pm

Leaving Heath at the hospital is so hard. As I was writing last night, I was reminded of all the prayers I have prayed for Heath's protection at work. I even remembered asking the Lord not to ask me to live this life without Heath. It hit me like a ton of bricks. God answered all of those prayers at once when He saved Heath's life.

"Lord, another day has come and gone. You have been my strength. You have held me up. You have allowed me to see the good. I know that Heath cannot remember a whole lot, but I pray for answers. This could be such a complicated situation, but I put it in your hands.

There are so many things that I don't know and so many questions that will arise over the coming days, but I ask you to protect Heath. Protect his name…his character…his reputation – protect him so that you might be glorified. May you be lifted high."

Later that night, thoughts were bouncing all over in my mind as I thought about our young children who were at home without us and how the Lord used people to love us.

Jan 31, 2021
11:50pm

I have made it back to the hotel. My body is so tired, but my mind is wide awake. There are so many people loving on us that I am absolutely moved to tears. Baskets of snacks, cards with such heartfelt words, people taking care of feeding my children and so many other acts of service. People are loving on us in every way imaginable and I am truly overwhelmed.

For the first couple of days in the hospital, Heath was taking some pretty strong stuff for pain and nerve issues, but he was always able to communicate with me and he seemed to think clearly for the most part.

Jan 31, 2021
11:55pm

Heath is in good spirits and he has had a pretty good day. He was able to sit in a chair for about 20 minutes today. He was able to move with some help to the side of the bed and sit with his feet off the side of the bed for 5-6 minutes today. His arm was less swollen, yet he still cannot feel anything. It seems like he may be having some pain or sensation in his hand that is nerve related. Oh, how I hope the Lord allows him to keep his hand, but he is at peace with losing it. In fact, he told one of the nurses this morning, he would gladly give them his hand if his buddy in the bed beside him could keep his other one.

Heath had a pretty hard time with an allergic reaction to whatever they used to wash the bed sheets. The only thing that really knocked him out was the Benadryl they gave him for the severe reaction he had to those bed sheets. Like…OUT…for a solid day and a half! He was sleeping with his mouth open and snoring, which he never does, and he had no clue what was going on. During the time I could not stay at the hospital, I went to the store and bought the cheapest set of twin sheets they had to offer and washed them with my laundry detergent at the hotel. As I suspected, after putting the new sheets under him, the breakout of his backside began to heal and the itching stopped almost immediately. So, thankfully, he was able to get off the Benadryl that took him to another world.

Several days after being admitted to the hospital and making sure everything was stable, 2 sweet, young girls came in our semi-private ICU room. They introduced themselves to us, one of them having a very thick accent from Trinidad. (We loved to hear her talk.) They explained that since the catheter had been removed and he was currently stable, they wanted to get a baseline for physical therapy. So, after taking some pain medication and with quite a bit of assistance, Heath was able to sit with his legs off the side of the bed.

The next day the young ladies brought some very nice-looking moon shoes with velcro straps. They had neither a right or left foot specifically and they were several inches too short for Heath's foot that normally wore a size 13 or size 14 shoe. However, after adding some extra padding to his soles and creatively strapping those shoes on his feet, he stood. Bearing all of his body weight on his charred, bandaged feet, he stood beside the bed for the first time since the accident. The next day, we strapped on his fancy shoes, put a belt around him and his blue hospital gown and helped him up onto his wounded feet. I watched (and videoed) as he slowly put one foot in front of the other. Steps. With a quiet determination, he inched out of the doorway towards the nurse's station. Slowly, but surely, he was walking under his own strength. As he returned to the room, tears streaming down my face, I was beaming with pride. He was going to beat this. I knew this man would fight and that he would never quit. This was only the beginning of a very long road ahead of us, but I knew he could do it if the Lord continued to allow him to live.

While he was sleeping one day, I sat beside his bed, thinking and praying. There were many times I wanted to open my eyes from this bad dream, but I was always reminded it was my reality. I have no idea how my Bible got to the hospital, but I needed hope and encouragement one day so I just started reading. As I read through the psalms, I came across Psalm 115:1 and it was as if the words I read were elevated off the page.

The verse reads, "Not to us, O Lord, not to us, but to your name be the glory because of your love and faithfulness." This was it. Because of God's love for me in sparing Heath's life and His faithfulness to lead me and prepare me, His name was to be lifted high. I was to give Him the glory for what He had done on my behalf. It was such a sobering thought that the Creator of the universe loved me and cared for me and even that He wanted what was best for me. There were times, especially in the beginning, where the Lord gave me quick reminders that He was in control and that nothing ever takes Him by surprise. This was one of those moments for me:

February 3, 2021
1:50am

Today has been a lot of thinking and reflecting. Heath had a tough day with therapy, but tough means good. He did great. It is really hard to understand how God could be working in so many different areas, but I got a text today that revealed to me God's true omniscience.

Heath was asked to record a single line of a poem several weeks ago. Several other people were also asked to record a different line of the poem. All of these recordings were put together to form an inspirational video that was shown a few hours before the accident.

Heath was asked to say this line:
"When you view what you think is the end."

I have watched the video several times since I received it today, but I still get chills when I hear it. What a reminder that our God is sovereign.

Our time in the ICU Burn unit only last about 5 days, but the crew behind that locked ICU door was phenomenal. Even though the nurses never really wanted to make me go, every night at 7pm, I had to leave the hospital, but I returned every morning at 8am. Those hours we were apart were difficult. I knew that it looked promising that Heath would ultimately live through this traumatic experience, but in the back of my mind, I knew he should not and I was subconsciously prepared in my heart for the bad news to come. I unknowingly anticipated his death every day. Without really being aware of the darkness that lurked in the back of my mind, I waited for the call from the doctor letting me know one of his organs was beginning to shut down. I knew there was no way for the doctors to evaluate the internal damage Heath may have suffered, so I steadied myself - thankful for the time I had each day, but always ready for it to quickly come to an end.

I had no idea at the time, but this was the beginning of my emotional withdrawal from Heath. My heart was building a wall around itself. The relationship we had built together was never perfect, but it was my sanctuary. He was the place where I could be completely who I am and where I could let go of my frustrations, my hurt, my anger and my pride. He believed in me. No matter what happened in our lives or what went wrong in the world, with my family, our kids, politics, or some crazy unforeseen tragedy, he was always my "right" no matter what in my life went "wrong." If I could get into his arms, he could make it right, not necessarily by doing anything specific, but instead by being my place of refuge. This time, however, my sanctuary was gone.

This attitude and the accident itself proved to be a very telling time in my life. It taught me where my heart truly was. My eyes were opened and the Lord allowed me to see, however, that my hope was in Heath and in his ability to care for me, rather than in the omnipotent Creator who formed me in my mother's womb. I learned why God gave me a man to help shelter me in times of tremendous pain and heartache, but I also began to understand more about myself. Most importantly though, I began to understand that in my weakness, I needed to learn how to lean on the Lord.

From the Hospital Bed

By: Heath Williamson

**This is a text message that Heath wrote
2 days after his accident to encourage our church.**

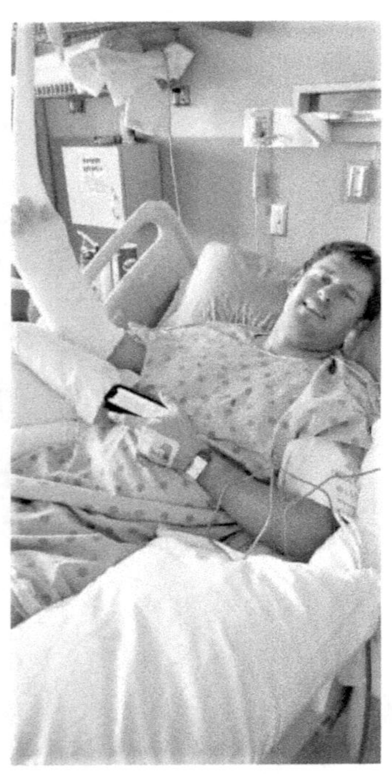

Good morning. I'm not sure how well this will turn out, but as I rest here this morning, I want so very badly to give an account of the goodness and mercy that God has shown to me. I can't wait to stand before you, but until then, maybe this will be an encouragement to you all.

Thursday afternoon somewhere around 4:00, in a bucket truck about 70 feet in the air, I was involved in an extremely high voltage electrical accident. I quickly thought about many things in those few short seconds, and I was so certain that my time here on earth was complete. I want you to know that in that moment, I was not fearful, but instead God overwhelmed me with His inexplicable peace. Just before I passed out, I mumbled "Michael, if you can hear me, this is it. I love the Lord my God and Rachel."

Sometime later, (I haven't been able to piece together exactly how many minutes passed), I began to come to and wake up. With the help of our coworkers, we were brought down to the ground. Several paramedics and two life flight helicopters were dispatched out to the job site. It is without a doubt, a MIRACLE, that God brought not only me, but Michael also through it.

I was able to walk off to the side and call Rachel, and believe it or not, lol, she answered. I don't even remember what I said exactly, but I needed to hear her voice and tell her that I loved her. I wanted her to know that I wasn't sure how things would turn out, but that I was at peace and I was going to be "ok." I could absolutely feel the peace in her voice as well.

With paramedics scurrying around us, I remember softly singing, "My hope is built on nothing less than Jesus' blood and righteousness." The paramedics loaded us into separate helicopters, a very tight squeeze I might add, and flew us to University Hospital in Mobile, AL, where they have been taking very good care of us and will continue to do so for some time.

Now, for my main reason in writing this: God chose to leave me here in my earthly role for a while longer. As I think about the earthly roles and responsibilities that God has given me: husband, father, son, brother, friend, co-worker, coach, and others, I have never been more committed to honoring God within these roles than I am right now. I will bless His name every day; I will praise His name forever and ever. My prayer is, that as you join me in considering God's amazing grace, mercy and faithfulness, that we can stir one another up towards love and good works. God has been so good to me, and I want to spend every day of the rest of my life being the ambassador of His truth, grace, mercy and love that He has called all of us to be. The gospel is simple.

"This is the record that God has given to us eternal life, and this love is in his Son. He that has the Son, has life, and he that has not the Son of God has not life. These things have I written unto you that you may believe in the name of the Son of God, that you may know that you have eternal life and that you may believe on the name of the Son of God." -1 John 5:11-13

I have a renewed passion and commitment to living out our faith together before a lost and dying world. I'm thankful for each one of you and the blessing that you are and have been to me and my family. Let your light so shine before men, that they may see your good works and glorify God, which is in heaven.

His Willing Vessel,
Heath

Chapter 8
In the Trenches

Be anxious for nothing, but in everything
by prayer and supplication, with thanksgiving,
let your requests be made known to God.
Philippians 4:6

I wrote to the Lord:

February 3, 2021
5:00am

"I don't even know how to pray or what to ask you for, but my eyes are on you. Spirit, intercede on my behalf. Ask the Father for what I need. Hold me up."

Almost daily, sometimes multiple times a day, I would hold the journal in my hands. Some of the pages are tear-stained, where I was pouring my heart out to the Lord. Some of them are songs that I was singing, reminding myself of truth. Many of the pages are prayers, but the majority of them were simply a release of the flood of emotions I felt from day to day. The range of those emotions was great. There were days I pleaded with the Lord for mercy, while I was also rejoicing in one of Heath's small victories. Those spiral-bound pages saw all of me:

the anger, the pain and some of the anticipated loss. I am still waiting for the rest of those emotions that are bottled up inside of me to surface. I wait, not so that I can wallow in the hurt, but so that I can accept it, close that chapter of my life and heal from it, with the hope that I can love Heath better and fully give myself to him again.

We were moved out of the ICU Burn Unit after being in there for 5 days. We were put on the 6th floor of the hospital where no one knew anything about our story. They had no idea what had happened to Heath 5 days earlier other than the few things they read in his chart. Every nurse or PCA that attended to Heath's needs, was equally as mesmerized with what had happened to Heath as the people were who took care of him in the ICU. There were many days when one of our nurses would bring several other nurses into our room just for us to give validation to the story.

We told as many people as would listen about the miracle we were living. I was still reluctant to believe that God would ultimately allow Heath to leave the hospital and go home to live life with us again, but I hoped with every fiber of my being that He would. The story was real. Sometimes when I tell it, it feels like I am telling a fairy tale, but it was my life. I actually lived it, but I had no way of knowing how God was going to end the story. Because of that, I continued to keep the wall around my heart.

I believe I put the wall there to lessen the blow of the pain I would experience if I were to lose Heath again. Thinking back, I can remember reasoning in my mind that unless the Lord came back in our lifetimes (which I believe is highly possible,) I had a 50/50 chance of reliving this loss again. Unless I died before him, I would feel these things again. Therefore, it was easier to refuse the butterflies and to reject the feelings of intimacy than to allow my heart to be recaptured by his love, only to have it stripped away again if things did not turn out as I hoped they would.

Hours began to turn into days and the days had become a full week.

Feb 3, 2021
11:05pm

"I have no idea how it is still Wednesday. All of the last 6 days have run together in my mind. My body is so tired, but my mind will not allow it to rest. The adrenaline rush of stopping dead in my tracks, flying to Mobile, looking into the eyes of my husband who should no longer be alive, sorting through calls and text, answering questions, along with other things is over. The rush is over but our time in the valley is not. And maybe I am wrong to call it a "valley" because it is truly one of the most wonderful things that has ever happened to me."

I missed the kids so much. I wanted to tell them everything, but I was afraid if they understood the gravity of the situation, they would pull away as well. I wanted them to cling to the hope of their daddy holding them again and coaching them again, even though the "facts" said it would never happen. In hindsight, I should have been more real with them.

The same God that was holding me was holding them as well. They have given me grace and they now understand all their daddy was up against when he was smiling at the camera as we were face-timing them. There were days I wanted to curl up in the hotel bed with all 6 of them, with no words said - which is impossible - and unleash all that I felt. I knew however, they would not understand the eruption of tears, nor did I know if I could stop once I allowed the dam to break. So, if the emotion could not be released through the ink of my pen, I held it all inside.

Feb 6, 2021
9:35am

We have been here around 8 days. I have not been able to sleep more than about 3 hours per night. I found some Tylenol PM in one of the bags and I was able to rest a little more last night. I just read the book of Ecclesiastes aloud while Heath was dozing.

"Now all has been heard;
Here is the conclusion of the matter.
Fear God and keep his commandments
for this is the whole duty of man."
"For God will bring every deed into judgment,
including every hidden thing,
whether it is good or evil."
Ecclesiastes 12:13-14 (NIV)

I read scripture aloud quite a bit. It was calming and peaceful in the stagnant air that encircled me. It was uplifting and gave my mind something to focus on rather than the tragedy. I learned to write verses on the mirror in the bathroom and in the thank you cards as I was writing. I wanted God's Word to be near to me. It helped my attitude and there were many times my attitude needed some major attention.

Feb 8, 2021
6:45am

The weekends at the hospital are slow. Heath has been in more pain, so he has slept more than he had been. I am feeling a little stir-crazy — already folded the rags and towels in the cabinet, rearranged the drinks and snacks again and repositioned the chair and table in the room. I want to go get some coffee and a shower, but I really don't want to leave even while he is sleeping. Once I get some more cards, I can go back to writing thank you notes. There are so many people that have loved us, I am truly overwhelmed.

Feb 9, 2021
11:45pm

I just finished writing cards to the kids. I cannot imagine how they are feeling, but I am looking forward to being in our own home, in our living room, with our kids all around us, talking with each other about all that God has done for us!!

Heath has surgery tomorrow. We are hoping to find that his body is responding well to the skin substitute, that there is no infection and that he is getting closer to being ready for skin grafts.

Feb 10
7:10am

They just took Heath to the operating room. The doctors and nurses didn't seem to be on the same page.

"Lord, please give him peace. Please strengthen Heath and hold him in your hands. Help them to get started quickly. Calm his nerves and give him peace in his spirit."

The doctors would typically call me halfway through the surgery if it was a long one, or call to tell me when the surgery was complete and Heath was in recovery. Those hours were long and the waiting seemed endless, but I busied myself with washing his bed sheet, gathering snacks he would enjoy and drinking far too much coffee. The call from the doctor was always appreciated, but if the news happened to be less than good, I was the one who would tell Heath how it went. Of course, they told him in the recovery room, but he was still waking up from the anesthesia, so he usually needed to be retold at least a couple of times.

Feb 10, 2021
9:25pm

We got a great report after Heath's surgery. The doctors said that his hand is getting blood from BOTH arteries and that blood is even getting to his fingers and thumb. What a blessing! Blood flow increases the chances of Heath being able to keep his hand. My heart praises the Lord.

The day was the best in my opinion. Heath was in good spirits. He pushed himself and I can tell he is getting ready to get back to the house. He was able to sit on the couch for awhile this evening. I think it was great for him to be out of the hospital bed.

The pain medicine Heath was on never "knocked-him-out." He could always carry on a conversation. He talked to different people on the phone, and he always sounded like the same 'ole man he had always been. But one of the pain medicines in particular, made him talk. And for me, this was pure bliss. I would wait about 30-45 minutes after they gave it to him, and I would go sit on the side of his bed. It was not long before the things in his heart would start coming out his mouth. I wish I had documented more things he said, so I could read them today. He is certainly a man of few words, so without medication, I hear very little from his heart of hearts.

Feb 11, 2021
11:45am

This has been a great morning!! Heath has felt good. I have been sitting in the corner of the room talking to him about all that God has done. He said that the men of the church are being stirred and the people of the community are loving on each other.

I told him this morning: I don't want people to just have warm, fuzzy feelings. I don't want them to see what God is doing and not come to know or feel him personally. I struggle with how to communicate it, but I want people to look beyond our situation, the love they have towards our family and wanting to help and actually "feel" what we are feeling. I want others to know peace in the midst of struggle and heartache.

Feb 12, 2021
2:30am

Heath is supposed to go back to the OR for the 4ᵗʰ time tomorrow. I think this time should be less aggressive, but they plan to look at this thumb and try to make a plan for doing a skin graft. He has a wound vac on his hand and his leg. Not sure if he will come back with them or not.

The kids are coming in the morning. Valentine's Day is Sunday so Heath sent me to Walmart to get stuffed animals and cards for the kids. Even though he is normally right-handed, he wrote all of the cards himself with his left hand and they were quite lengthy cards. So precious.

I remember around the time of these journal entries reading a quote from a card someone sent to us. It read, "Sometimes God may allow hardships to reach us so that His mercy can reach beyond us." There have been many times that I have read a quote or saying like that and skimmed right over it, but those words penetrated my heart. His mercy was capable of reaching even beyond what I needed. Simple reminders of truth – God's truth – seemed to find their way into my life.

Feb 15, 2021
4:05pm

Heath just came back from surgery a little while ago. He is struggling to come back from the anesthesia. He has done this once before. A little scary. The burn doctor who did the surgery was very encouraged. Today is the first time he has seen new growth around Heath's thumb. His next surgery is scheduled for Friday.

Feb 17, 2021
12:00pm

Been reading in Daniel. The note in my study bible says this for Daniel 6:21-23: The person who trusts in God and obeys his will is untouchable until God takes him. To trust God completely is to have immeasurable peace.

We have family friends that live in Mobile, and they allowed me to have things mailed to their house. Cards came in the mail to the hospital and to their house as well. The encouragement we received was overwhelming. People that I had never met were praying for my husband. We were so humbled.

Feb 19, 2021
9:15pm

Today has been a rough day for me emotionally. I have struggled with whether or not I trust the Lord. I know what is right in my head and I want to act on it, but I struggle to feel the right things in my heart.

The adrenaline rush of the last 3 weeks has been crazy. Very little sleep, tons of coffee, more sugar than I have eaten in the last 2 years, fast food every day, but I have come down off the rush (or I think I have).

Every time Heath brushes my hands or wants to kiss my face, I feel the tingle of the butterflies, but my heart says "no." "Don't do it. Don't reattach. The pain will be too much if you really lose him." I can bathe him, help him change, keep up with his medication, kiss him – basically everything a nurse would do (except the kiss), but it is just "what I do." It feels cold somehow.

I have busied myself with blessing nurses with snack bags, writing thank you notes, cleaning and rearranging the room and making runs for lunch or supper. I am not mad or upset. Not angry or mad. I just kind of feel nothing at all.

I guess as I think back to the night in the ER, I had prepared myself for Heath to die. Even if he made it through surgery, surely his organs were cooked on the inside. They could never work properly again. Even though I was relieved to get the call that night saying he made it through the surgery, my heart still didn't relax. And I think I still feel that way at times. I push back the butterflies almost as if I am fighting myself. I cannot surrender myself again. Any form of intimacy is directly connected to my heart. It is almost as if I have built a wall of defense around my own heart against my own husband. I want to tear it down and I have tried to ignore it, but I don't know how. Very strange feeling.

"Lord God, I want to be honest with you. I don't want to fake it. I don't want to hide behind 'happiness' or 'everything is just going to work out.' I want to be real. I want to see myself as you see me and I want my heart to cry out to You. Help my heart to trust so that I can believe you have really given him back to me. Help me to live in the moment. Help me give my heart back to Heath. Why would I want to keep it? If I knew he would be gone tomorrow, I would want to give him all that I am. Why would I pretend? Why am I withholding my heart? Help me to embrace the butterflies. Thank you for loving me and thinking of me when you saved his life."

I went to church with my aunt and uncle that still live in Mobile a few times. The worship services were exactly what my heart needed to be encouraged. I looked forward to being there and just being reminded of God's truth. I wanted to think about the right things. I wanted to be obedient to the Lord, but my flesh was so weak. I felt like Peter. In my mind, I was sold out, but when the rubber met the road, I was climbing an uphill battle, clinging to the Lord as my only source of strength.

Feb 26, 2021
3:15pm
Daddy came to see me. I needed the encouragement from him so much. The Lord is at work behind the scenes. I do not have to understand what He is doing to be obedient.

We are trying to manage Heath's pain after surgery. The nerve pain especially is rough.

Mar 3, 2021
9:45am

Heath is in surgery now. We are hoping he is ready for a skin graft on his left foot and possibly his wrist. God has been so gracious. Watching the wound care team change his dressing yesterday reminded me again that Heath even being alive is a miracle. Whether they are able to save his right hand or not, we still do not know. Such a strange and bittersweet feeling. Either way though, he will need to learn to do things a new way and he will.

Some of our closest friends came to see me one day around the first of March. I had been battling in my mind how to approach Heath and his road to recovery. I am a realist. I did not want to have unrealistic expectations, but I also wanted to trust that the Lord was capable of healing Heath completely if He chose to do so. Because of this quandary, I struggled with how to love and support Heath on his road to recovery.

After a long conversation under the covered awning of the hospital that day, I am convinced that God allowed those friends to come into my life at the perfect time. I was low. Very low. I needed reminding that Heath needed me to swing for the fences with him. Our life together had already been good, but even through all of this, it was going to get better. It may have been that day alone that truly shaped my perspective for the future.

March 3, 2021
11:10am

I just talked to the burn doctor. Heath is out of surgery. To this point we have really had no setbacks, but the surgery today seemed to be just that. Heath has some infection in his wrist. The tendons in his wrist that were once attached have deteriorated and are no longer attached. This would explain why he cannot rotate his wrist or move his thumb at all.

March 4, 2021
9:15am
We have spent a good bit of time talking about whether it would be better to have the hand God gave Heath that won't do what he needs it to do and that can't feel anything, or would it be better to take it off and hope that a prosthetic would give him a better quality of life.

"Lord my heart can't do it. I am about to break under the pressure. The road ahead is going to be long no matter what, but I cannot be responsible for these kinds of decisions. Please don't ask me to decide. Please let the doctors do it."

March 5, 2021
3:15pm
Wound care today was awful. When they uncovered Heath's arm, I was not prepared for what I would see. He is going back to the OR tomorrow. We really don't know how much more of his wrist they will have to take.

It is hard to understand how saving Heath's hand is even still on the table. Literally, over half his wrist is gone. They took all the tendons, one of the two arteries and only one main nerve is left.

"Lord, the days ahead are so uncertain. My heart is still fearful at times. Even though you miraculously saved Heath's life, will I lose him still? Help me to trust you – in the good and in the bad."

For several days my mind was heavy with the weight of the

decisions ahead. I had moved my little couch on wheels over beside Heath's bed. We joked that it was a hospital-grade king sized bed. It was nowhere close to awesome, but at least we could touch each other. There were a lot of nights that Heath didn't sleep much. I thought he was dreaming, but he could never remember the next morning.

I continued to call out to the Lord for help. I wanted the best for Heath, but I wanted to go home. I missed the kids so much. It was like I had a huge hole in my heart. The pain in my jaw and at the base of my neck was so bad at times. I knew the stress that was mounting on my shoulders was the source of my physical pain, but I was not sure what to do about it.

March 5, 2021
4:20pm

Today has been a hard day, but a good day. During Heath's surgery this morning, I left the hospital. The weight of the surgery was so heavy. As I was driving by Dauphin Way Baptist Church, right off the interstate, I could hear the chimes playing from the steeple of the church. I rolled my window down so that I could hear the bells and the words of the song came flooding my heart.

I pulled into the church parking lot as tears began to stream down my face. Although I could not sing with my voice, my heart was crying out to the Lord as I sang along with the bells the old hymn How Great Thou Art. The tears were falling. Release. Finally. They came.

There were a lot of tears that day, but I think the Lord began to teach me that I can cry without being angry or frustrated. I can simply cry as a release of emotion. I told the Lord I don't know how to pray or what to say, but I want to trust him regardless of whether Heath is able to keep his hand or not – whether he "lives" or not.

That was such a powerful day in my walk with the Lord. God used the bells of that church to allow my heart to feel His closeness. It was as tangible as though He had placed his hand on my shoulder. I knew He was there. As close as my next breath. It was a reminder that I was not alone. Ponder for a moment, if you will, the words of that hymn:

How Great Thou Art

(Verse 1)
O Lord my God, when I in awesome wonder
Consider all the world Thy hands have made
I see the stars, I hear the rolling thunder
Thy power throughout the universe displayed

(refrain)
Then sings my soul, my Savior God to Thee
How great Thou art, How great Thou art
Then sings my soul, my Savior God to Thee
How great Thou art, How great Thou art!

(Verse 3)
And when I think, that God His Son not sparing
Sent Him to die, I scarce can take it in
That on the cross, my burden gladly bearing
He bled and died to take away my sin

(Verse 4)
When Christ shall come, with shouts of acclamation
And take me home, what joy shall fill my heart
Then I shall bow, in humble adoration
And then proclaim: My God how great Thou art!

It gives me chills today just writing it down! It truly was a reminder that even though so much is going wrong, the Lord was to be magnified and lifted high. It reminded me of this scripture in Ecclesiastes 7:14:

"When times are good, be happy; but when times are bad, consider: God has made the one as well as the other." (NIV)

Valentine's Day

by: Maci Williamson

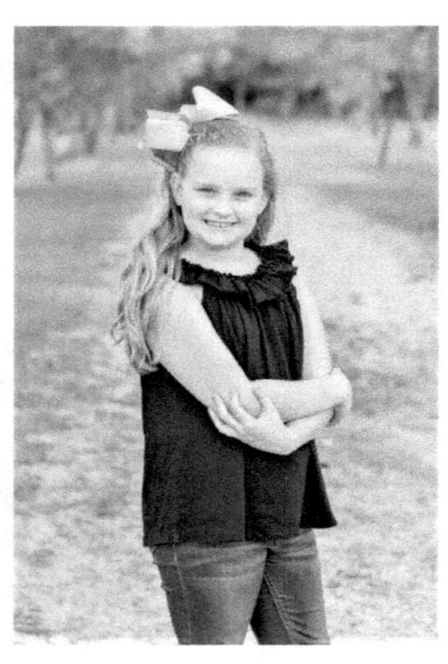

Valentine's Day while Mom and Dad were in the hospital was hard for me. I remember waking up Valentine's morning in the pajamas Mom sent to me earlier in the week. My grandmother, who we call Babo, had a little gift bag for my brother, my sisters and me. The bag said "Love." I opened the gift and it was from my daddy. There was a small stuffed animal, a pack of Reese's candy and a card. I opened the red envelope. The card had a little bear on the front holding a bouquet of balloons. Tears began to fall from my face as I started reading the words my daddy wrote to me. Daddy was right-handed before his accident, but he could no longer use his right hand.

With his left hand, Daddy wrote, *I love you, Maci Kate. YOU ARE BEAUTIFUL.* My tears covered the card. I felt so loved.

I was so ready for Mom and Dad to come home. I had so many feelings I did not know what to say or what to do. It was a Valentine's Day I will never forget.

Chapter 9
Back to the Drawing Board

It is good for a man to bear the yoke in his youth.
Lamentations 3:27 (NIV)

After a good month and a half into our hospital stay, neither one of us knew what day of the week it was, what time of the day it was, or whether it was day or night. Most of all, we both missed our bed and our children. Everyone told me I would lose track of time while we were in the hospital, but since I am typically really good with a planner, I did not believe it. I could not understand how I could lose a day of the week in my mind altogether. But…it happened.

I continued to journal, and Heath continued to go back to the operating room for one reason or another. He was such a valiant warrior. It was incredible to watch his resilience. There is NO possible way on the planet I could have physically gone through all that he endured. No way.

For a long time, I was the only one allowed to visit Heath in the hospital and that was very hard for me. I felt tremendous guilt that his parents, nor our children could see one of the most important people in their lives. It troubled me to the point that I wrote letters to the administrators of the hospital, to the governor, and to a radio station that Heath frequently listened to. A lot was going on in our world at the time that struck fear in the hearts of people like never before, but the rules and regulations put in place, were hindering people from healing emotionally.

Thankfully, a few weeks into our hospital stay, the governor changed one of the regulations allowing an additional visitor to come into the hospital. This meant that Heath was finally able to see his parents. What a blessing that was! In the meantime, our burn doctor was phenomenal and continued to work through Heath's unique situation. He brought in a plastic surgeon and another surgeon that specialized in hands to help him formulate a new plan for Heath. We had spent a full 6 weeks in the hospital and were hoping to be finished with surgeries and be back home with our kids, but now we were back to the drawing board.

My journaling became more routine as the days passed. I almost used it as a way to keep up with time, surgeries, people I met, and scriptures that I was reading or studying.

March 9, 2021
8:00 pm

Heath is sleeping. He left for surgery today around 12:15 pm and did not get back into the room until about 5 pm. His feet are ready to graft, but since we are going to be here waiting for his hand, wrist, and calf, they have decided to see how much his feet will heal on their own. The hand surgeon thinks that the muscle in Heath's arm looks good enough to try a tendon transfer. We are looking at next Tuesday for that surgery. Wow. A week. With basically no progress.

March 11, 2021
1:20pm

Very thankful to be in the hospital room with Heath today. He struggled after coming back from surgery. The combination of the anesthesia and the pain medicine was too much. At 2:30 am, he was making old school buses into homes for homeless children, and he was heading outside to get some sun. At some point, he was afraid to eat a Cliff bar because I had intentionally rubbed it on the floor to contaminate it, but he was altogether cute as pie while he was talking out of his mind. I was able to keep the nurses from giving him a double dose of the pain medication and I was thankful to be here to see the funny stuff.

The days were so long. It seemed that we were always waiting just to wait some more. I am not sure why the weekends were the worst. It always seemed like nothing really happened. The main doctors were not there and unless there was a true emergency, we just had to wait until Monday. The monotone voice that came across the PA system day in and day out announcing – Trauma Alert to the Emergency Room, Trauma Alert to the Emergency Room – was chilling. Also, the feeling of the wind from the life-flight helicopters as they landed on the helipad sent my mind back to the day my life changed forever. Just a few weeks back, my husband was "the" *Trauma Alert to the Emergency Room,* and he was flown onto that same helipad. That was the night I thought I would lose him to death. Sheeeew. Such hard memories.

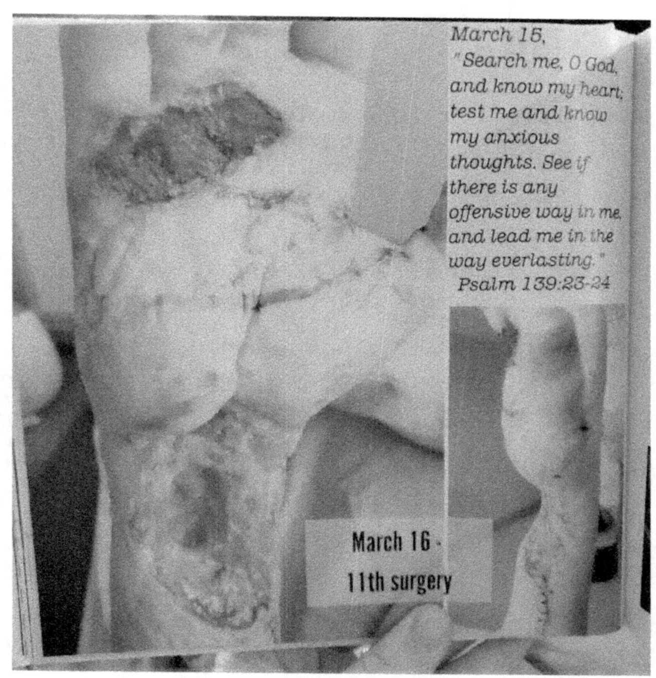
March 16,
"Search me, O God,
and know my heart;
test me and know
my anxious
thoughts. See if
there is any
offensive way in me,
and lead me in the
way everlasting."
Psalm 139:23-24
March 16 -
11th surgery

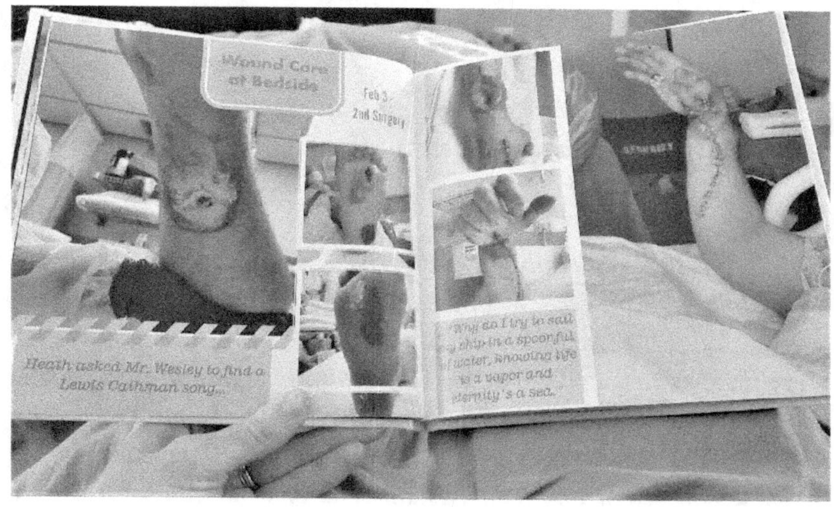
Wound Care
at Bedside
Feb 3 -
2nd Surgery
Heath asked Mr. Wesley to find a
Lewis Cathman song...
Why so I try to sail
a ship in a spoonful
of water, knowing life
is a vapor and
eternity's a sea.

March 22, 2021
3:05 pm

Heath is asleep. I am listening to a praise and worship playlist a friend made for me. Surgery for the hand reconstruction is scheduled for tomorrow morning. My heart is expectantly heavy. The stakes are very high. We do not know if there is enough of his hand still alive to proceed or what the outcome of the surgery will be.

"Do not be anxious about anything, but in everything, by prayer and petition, with thanksgiving, present your requests to God. And the peace of God, which transcends all understanding, will guard your hearts and minds in Christ Jesus." -Philippians 4:6-7

March 23, 2021
5:55 am

The lab woke us up at 4:30 am. They cannot draw his blood because Heath has a central line in his neck. Of course, I can't go back to sleep. Our nurse started a bag of fluids and drew the blood they needed from the line.

Not sure if I am just more uptight than I realize or what, but I feel so distant from Heath. I have felt this way for a couple of days. Not sure what is up, but I am asking the Lord to work.

"Lord, this is a really big day. I have been calling out to You. I know that you can heal Heath's hand, but even if you choose not to, I trust You. I will still magnify your name. My "request" …my "petition" is that you allow the tendons in his hand to be alive and capable of sustaining the tendon transfer. Please go before the doctor and nurses. Prepare the way for them. Use them. God, I am asking you to show yourself strong today. Thank you for what you have already done on our behalf. Thank you for saving Heath. Thank you for *growing me and stretching me. You are a good, good Father."*

Like it was yesterday I can remember sitting in a small coffee shop around the corner from the hospital for several hours anticipating the call from the doctor saying that Heath had made it through the 8-hour surgery. They called in one doctor to harvest a portion of Heath's hamstrings in his left leg and another doctor to then attach it to the muscle below his elbow and then to his palm. Because there was so little blood flow in Heath's arm and hand, the plastic surgeon cut a "flap" in Heath's stomach and sewed his arm to the flap. This meant that for 3 weeks Heath's arm was sewn to his stomach and could not be removed. This allowed the blood from his stomach to promote the blood flow and "healing" for his arm, wrist, and hand.

March 23, 2021
7:15 pm
I am sitting in the hospital waiting for Heath to come back from surgery. They were able to do the hand reconstruction. The Lord heard me and He answered me. I want to cry so badly, but the tears just won't come.

The prayer of my heart was that the tendons left in his hand would be alive enough to do the surgery, AND THEY WERE!! The specialized hand surgeon was also able to remove a ton of scar tissue. The scar tissue is what was keeping Heath from being able to rotate his arm toward his face. Heath's hand will be attached to his stomach for 3 weeks, but nothing is binding his arm in place but an Ace wrap. Not sure how this will go or how I will keep him from "jerking" in the night and separating it. Pretty nervous.

March 25, 2021
8:00 pm

Not exactly sure why the day has been so hard. I feel heavy somehow. Knots in my stomach and I feel so distant from Heath. Not very many butterflies to embrace lately. I hope things will get better when we get home, but I know there will be so much going on. I am scared that I will grow completely cold.

Heath had another surgery or 2 cleaning up his right leg and preparing his feet to be grafted. The itching and oozing of his arm were constant and the sheer determination to "keep it still" was emotionally exhausting. The raw flesh that was exposed under a thin layer of bandages that I changed daily was a hard thing for both of us to see, but his will to conquer the task before him was indomitable.

April 4, 2021
2:25 pm

Easter Sunday. This certainly has not been an "Easter" that you typically think of. We watched the Sunrise Service from our church back home thanks to a close friend. We listened to some music and worshiped together for an hour or so. Then, I went to the local church that I have been attending while we have been here. Heath watched the service live from the hospital while I was there.

It was a great day until I got back to the hospital. Several things happened that caused our minds and hearts to be distracted from who God is and what this day means for us as believers.

I miss the kids so much. Sometimes I wish I would wake up from a bad dream. Is this my life?? Is this really a part of God's will for my life?? What am I supposed to do in this hospital room where my hands are tied and I am COMPLETELY out of control?? My questions come out of a grateful and sincere heart. I am aware of God's goodness. I know and understand what my life "should" look like today, but the Lord was merciful to me.

"Now, Lord, what do I do with all of this? What do I do with the testimony you have given us?"

Heath had yet another surgery to clean out more dead tissue and muscle and to see if his leg and his feet were ready for the skin grafts. Several things happened between the time they took him for surgery and the time they called to tell me he was in recovery. Those things that happened produced anger and rage in me that I have never known, and I hope to never experience again. For fear of sounding controversial, I will not share the details of the story, but I will say that I was asked to leave the hospital immediately and was asked to take with me all the stuff I had accumulated over our 10-week stay. In addition, I was not allowed to see my husband once he came out of surgery.

April 7, 2021
10:10 am
I have so much anger, frustration, and anxiety my heart may explode!! I know I should speak as little as possible because with ALL the emotion I have, I will say something I should not.

"Oh Lord, I need you. Why do you have me here…alone…in a hotel room? I need to know that you are still here. I feel so confused. Is this really a part of your plan? I do not want to be like the Israelites grumbling in the wilderness after all you had done for them. I want to be like Daniel, fearless before the king."

As I found myself, alone and confused in that hotel room, I cried out to the Lord in an audible voice. I did not shout, but I was probably close to it. "What am I doing here!?! Answer me. If you will just tell me what to do, I will do it, but I cannot just sit here!"

In the silence of that lifeless hotel room, obviously, he did not answer me aloud. But in frustration, I threw myself across the bed with my Bible. Pouting, I opened up randomly to the book of Lamentations where we read about the mercies of the Lord being new every morning. I read Lamentation 3:27, which says, "It is good for a man to bear the yoke while he is young." I read it several times, cross-referenced it, and pondered it.

The notes in my Bible at the bottom of the page said this:

To *"bear the yoke"* means to willingly come under God's discipline or correction and to learn what He wants to teach you. This involves the following: (1) Silent reflection on what God wants (2) Repentant humility (3) Self-control in the face of adversity (4) Confident patience, depending solely on the divine Teacher to bring about loving lessons in our lives for our good.

Once again, he answered me. Oh, my goodness. How hard it was to humble myself when I was right and they were wrong. I wanted to scream from the rooftops, but I allowed my emotions and zeal for the truth to get out of control. The Lord, however, graciously called me back to Himself, in addition to removing me from the hospital so I did not get myself put in jail. After a day and a half, the hospital allowed me to go back in to see Heath. Reluctantly, I went.

April 8, 2021
7:15 am

Heath made it to a room last night at about 6 pm. He was hungry so I picked up Zaxby's and went to the hospital even though I didn't want to go. I think I slept an hour in total. I was still awake at 1:30 am…meds at 2 am…vitals at 3:15 am…more meds/vitamins at 5 am…blood drawn at 5:30 am. And here I am.

I need a cup of coffee, but because I was kicked out of the hospital, I don't have any of my stuff, including my coffee pot and my cute little mini frig for my half and half. I just have a bad attitude and I know it. Oh good…more vitals at 7:30 am. I guess I will just get up and clean the room… again.

The 3 weeks of waiting for Heath's arm to heal enough to detach it from his stomach came to an end around the second week of April. Heath was advocating for us to go home, but as badly as I wanted to see the kids, I did not want to go home. I had so much emotion built up that I had no idea what to do, and I knew diving right back into life was *not* what I needed to do. All I wanted was to snuggle down in my bed with my children and cry. But…if you have children, you know that cannot happen without lots of tossing and turning, giggling and fighting and a ton of questions from the small people. Heath could not understand my viewpoint at all. He needed his kids, so he continued to push for the discharge papers.

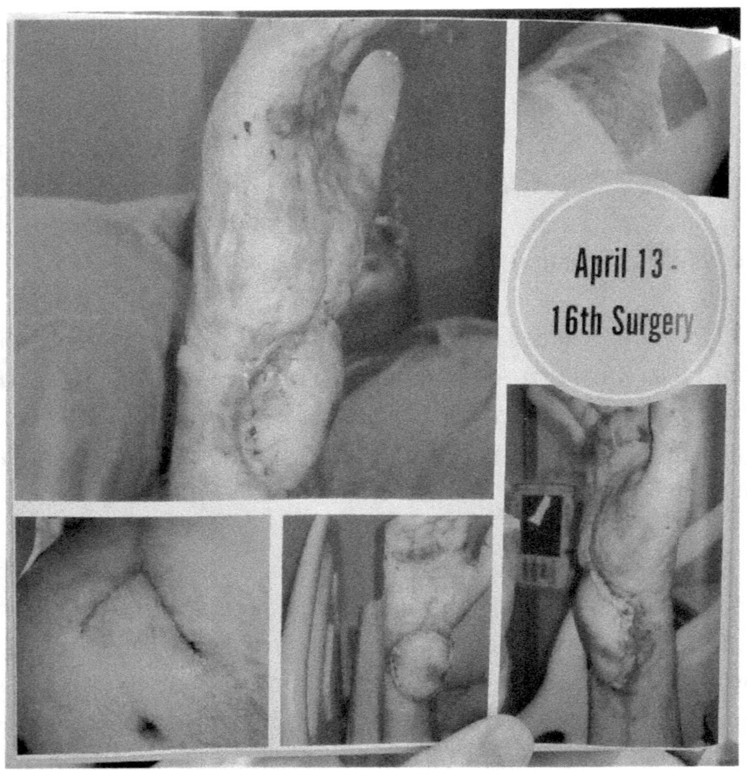

April 13, 2021
7:50pm

I am waiting for Heath to come from the Operating Room. This has been surgery number 16 since January 28th. His hand is no longer sewn to his stomach even though he doesn't know it yet. I think it is very feasible for us to go home in a couple of days, but I don't know. We will wait on see how wound care and physical therapy go tomorrow.

April 14, 2021
8:30 pm

I am not sure how I feel about going home. I need a couple of days. Life certainly has not slowed down at home just because we were not there to live it. My chest is so tight and at times I feel like my heart may explode.

I am so thankful and overwhelmed…for all the people that have worked at the house…money people have sent to help us…people that have kept our grass cut…people that have taken food to feed our kids…and so many other little things that I could go on for days naming.

"Lord, you have been so good to us. You have loved us beyond measure …so much more than we deserve…and your blessings continue to flow. And while I am thankful, my tank is so empty. I am literally running on fumes. I don't know if I even have enough left in the tank to get us home.

"I want to hold the kids. I hope they can help me cry. I really think I need to cry. Not sure exactly what the answer is, but real life is about to happen whether I want it to or not. My safety bubble is almost gone. You know I'm scared and I'm tired. You know that I am weak – in my body and in my mind. Please help me."

We were finally discharged from the hospital. Heath was able to breathe in the fresh air and feel the sun on his face again. We both still had a very long road ahead of us and we both had a good bit of healing that needed to be done. We were both thankful for the opportunity to see our six, beautiful children and to lie down together in our big, king-sized bed.

Looking Back

By: Allyx Williamson

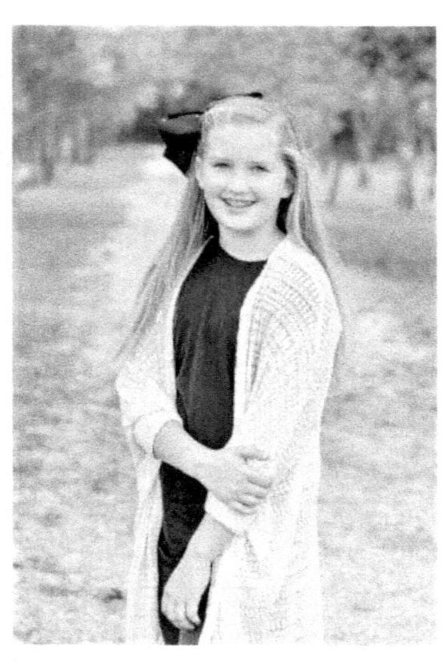

Mom asked me to write down some of my thoughts about dad's accident. I will start by telling you that I am not a patient person. I like to "be in the know." I like to know what is happening…to know where we will be going…to know what we will be doing. When Mom first got word about the accident, my world was flipped upside down. I felt very scattered and confused. None of us knew any details or what the next day would hold.

Several weeks later, while my parents were still in the hospital, I can remember sitting at my grandmother's house reading cards I had received from friends and family and a few cards Mom had sent. I can still remember some of my thoughts from that day so vividly. *I don't understand. Why did this happen? Are Mom and Dad ever coming home? Will we all ever be all together again?* And of course, I thought about dad. *Would he make it through the next surgery? Would he lose his right hand? Will he ever coach my softball team again? Will he be there to walk me down the aisle when I get married?*

My life seemed so unsure. Everything seemed "up in the air." Anytime we went to see Mom and Dad at the hospital, I could hardly wait to get there. But then when we had to leave, the thought of knowing how long it would be before we could go back was so hard.

Through all the hard days, God was good to me. He was with me on the days I wished my life could "go back to normal." He was there when I asked, "Why does it have to be this way?" He was never caught by surprise, and I was never alone. He was with me during all the hard times following dad's accident. Every step of the way, God had a plan and He was using Dad's situation to bring Himself glory.

Chapter 10
The Trial Continues

The Lord is my light and my salvation;
whom shall I fear?
The LORD is the strength of my life;
of whom shall I be afraid?
Psalm 27:1

We had been out of the hospital a few days, but Heath still had at least 2 surgeries ahead of him. I was a basket-case and had no idea if I was coming or going. I literally lived minute to minute.

April 22, 2021
3:30 am

We have been home for 6 days now. Honestly – it seems like an eternity. I feel like I am as slow as a turtle and like everyone is running circles around me. We have A LOT of "readjusting" to do but with the Lord's help, I believe we can do it.

As I write this chapter, I am sitting in the same local coffee shop that is just around the corner from the hospital that I visited numerous times during our hospital stay. It has a quaint little prayer room tucked away in the back of it. There is a beautiful stained-glass door that separates the prayer room from the rest of the coffee shop. It has a calming and soothing atmosphere, which is aided by worship music playing throughout the building. The walls are decorated solely with scripture and simple reminders of truth. Because I struggled immensely to take my thoughts completely captive while Heath remained in the hospital and through the many surgeries he had before we were discharged, this little coffee shop was my place of refuge. After leaving Heath at the hospital for surgery this morning, even with the numbness in my soul, I could feel the presence of the Lord when I walked through the door. I was able to remind myself of the truth, rather than dwelling in fear and allowing the anxiety from the enemy to take hold of me.

Currently, I am holding a hot cup of Columbian roast with just enough cream to turn the color of the coffee blonde. It was served to me in a white coffee mug that fits perfectly in my hand. Just the warmth of the cup in my hand allows me to relax so I can think and ponder. I really cannot explain the peace I feel. Perhaps it is because of the vivid memories of my time here while we were in the hospital or thinking back on all the prayers I prayed for Heath in this very building. Maybe it is just the presence of the Lord, the scriptures on the walls or the music in the background, but here I can open my heart. It is in this coffee shop that I can continue mending together the broken pieces of my heart. I can reflect…contemplate. No one needs my conversation. No chores to be done. Nothing needs my immediate attention. This certain quietness allows my struggles and my fears to come to the surface and it gives me the desire to be completely vulnerable.

It is here that I become aware of what is truly inside of me…aware of the fear and doubt that I continue to hold captive in my heart…aware of the feelings that I have buried deep within me…aware of the anger that haunts me while I sleep. God is teaching me that when these emotions are allowed to rise to the surface, that they can be removed. As I sit here, I am allowed to be completely real with myself and know that my Heavenly Father sees me where I am. I can be reminded that He has carried me through the physical pain I have felt because of the lack of sleep. He has shouldered the weight of my emotional pain from the anticipated loss of my husband. He has eased the separation anxiety I felt being away from my kids. This reminder alone is proof that He will see me through to the other side.

As I embrace the freedom to reflect this morning, I have considered the number of people we have come to know as a result of Heath's accident. Even the staff in the outpatient surgery department called Heath by name as he entered the waiting room this morning and Heath remembered them too. He remembered what town they grew up in, where they went to high school and what football team they will be pulling for. So many unique relationships that the Lord has used to bless us in ways they may never even comprehend! Hopefully, we are nearing the end of our "surgical journey," as he is currently undergoing his twentieth surgery since the accident this morning. We have no idea whether the Lord will choose to give him back the function of his right hand or not, but with thankfulness for what God has already done, that is my prayer and petition to Him. Whether He chooses to answer me the way I want Him to or not, I know he is capable of working another miracle on our behalf. One doctor told us while we were still in the hospital that Heath would never drive a nail with a hammer, hit a baseball, or swing a golf club again, but I know God can work beyond all that we can ask or imagine. I choose, however, to trust Him either way - in life or in death...in complete healing or not...in comfort or in struggle.

My desire is to be surrendered to the will of God, confidently knowing that He holds the future, and He knows what is best for me, for Heath, and for our family. Therefore, I have peace. It is, however, a different peace than some people think of, I believe. This peace is not a result of good things happening or the absence of conflict and pain. It is neither a result of turning over a new leaf or of intentional, positive thinking. This peace is knowing that God is in control of my life and of my circumstances and nothing happens to me that He does not allow.

When I have a few moments to myself, I like to look back through my journal just to remind myself that I did really live in a hospital a few days short of 3 months and to remember the way I felt during our time there. Seeing my written words reminds me that the events which I have written about are real. Those things actually happened to the man I love and I did experience hurt, pain, anger, and fear as a result of it. But the chicken scratch in that spiral-bound notebook is part of who I am and it serves as a reminder of what God has done for me. Day after day...week after week...and ultimately month after month, He gave me supernatural strength that was absolutely beyond who I am as a person.

There were days when I just knew that my physical body could not go on without more rest. There were days I could only eat rice and grits because stress had caused my jaw to clench down so tightly that it was too painful to chew, but He provided. He sustained me when I felt nauseated for days at a time. He gave me breath when my chest was so tight, I found it difficult to breathe. Somehow the Lord stilled the anxiousness of my heart when I turned to Him because there certainly were days when I found it easier to flounder around in my circumstances than to look to the Lord for answers. But the Lord was gracious to me as He taught me to depend on Him.

"Dependence" on the Lord is not a verb that lacks action. When one finds themselves "dependent," they must choose to lay down what seems right and fair and they must ask, seek and plead with the Lord. Does the Lord need us to ask anything of Him? Does he need me to ask Him to meet my needs? Of course not. Be we need it. I need it. My dependence on the Lord has deepened with each day of this journey. I have learned to consciously step aside, to peacefully remind myself of truth, and to actively trust Him; therefore, even as hard as it has been to go through, I am thankful for this journey.

There is more "growing" ahead for me to do, but I am confident that the arms of the Lord will carry me through the storms as they come. Just as James mentioned in his letter to the first-century Christians, the question is not "if" the trials will come, but rather "when" they come. The thought has come to my mind numerous times over the last few months – this "trial" will not be my last.

As I mentioned in the beginning pages of this book, my goal has never been to glorify the accident that we lived through, nor to elevate anything within us. It was and is instead, to point people to the cross. My objective in reliving the events of the past 9 months myself and then choosing to tell you, as a friend would tell a friend, is simply to give you hope and encouragement that our God is real. He is the same miracle-working God today that we read about in the stories of the Old Testament.

We have read in Sunday School about the mouths of lions being shut for the entirety of the night while Daniel waited for morning to come. We read to our children about Moses parting the Red Sea through the power of God and the people walking through the sea on dry ground. He is the same God who worked miracles through the apostles in the New Testament to give validity to what they were preaching, which was that Jesus was the only way to the Father. That simple truth is still true today. The end of this life is drawing near. No man knows the day or the hour of our Lord's return, nor do we know if the Lord will allow us to wake up tomorrow with breath in our lungs. But God is still the same - yesterday, today, and forever – and He longs to have a relationship with each one of us. He created every person on purpose and with a purpose – no exceptions.

I think the analogy of Heath and his brother enjoying the day and putting off "the chores" or the things of importance to the very end is where many people stand spiritually. Some people are subconsciously choosing to live life the way they want to live it and when they have lived a full life, they plan to turn over a new leaf and start "living right." Some never miss a Sunday at church but find themselves hypocritically only going through the motions. Others may have never seen the inside of a church building other than for a wedding or a funeral. Regardless of where we find ourselves in life, the "need" is the same for all people from every walk of life. We all need a relationship with God the Father and that relationship is only available through the blood shed by Jesus Christ. There is no one righteous, no, not one. It does not matter who you are or where you have been, the Bible says in Isaiah 59 that "the Lord's hand is not shortened, that it cannot save."

It is the cry of God's heart that all men come to faith in Him, but the Bible is clear that no man can come to the Father unless the Spirit draws him. What if the Holy Spirit has used words on the pages of this book to prick your heart? What if God calls your heart through a sermon at church or something you hear on the radio? How sad it would be for one to know the Spirit is calling him and to reject the call on his life, yet not live long enough to be called again. The result of doing so would mean total separation from our Creator in hell for all eternity.

My plea is that if you have never acknowledged your need

for forgiveness and asked the Lord to save your life that you would not wait another day...another hour...another minute to confess your sin and ask the Lord to save you. The gospel is simple. "If you confess with your mouth, Jesus is Lord, and believe in your heart that God raised him from the dead, you will be saved." Sometimes we make it so complicated, but the fact is anyone who calls on the name of the Lord will be saved. In a world full of doubt, distrust, and despair, this simple truth is a breath of fresh air. And for some, it may be a truth that you have never been confronted with before.

Heath had placed his trust in the Lord to save him when he was only 9 years old. He had no idea where his life would take him, but even at such a young age, he recognized that he was a sinner in need of forgiveness. Even though he was seemingly "the perfect child", he was not enough, relying on himself alone. He needed the blood of Jesus to cover his sins. As the song says I learned in Vacation Bible School as a child...*I have decided to follow Jesus - no turning back, no turning back*. Heath chose to follow Jesus with his life. He lived a life that was *not* perfect, but he was characterized by following the Lord and it allowed him to build relationships of trust with the people he interacted with on a daily basis.

It was that one choice to trust in and follow Jesus that brought about the unmistakable peace Heath had when he closed his eyes in what he thought was certain death...on the 28th day of January - 2021...in the middle of a field...70 feet in the air...with absolutely no warning. If God had not chosen to step in, Heath would be in heaven with his Savior today. And because of his relationship with the Lord at his time of death, I would have been able to live the rest of my life knowing I would see him again.

For there will be a day when I too will close my eyes in death and awaken in heaven with our Creator, as a result of placing my faith and trust in Jesus Christ alone. BUT… praise the Lord with me for HIS intervention! I will be able to live the rest of my life with the peace and confirmation that God is real, knowing that IF *January 28, 2021, had been his last day on this earth,* I would see him again. Oh, but what a mighty God we serve!! HE CHOSE in his mercy to spare Heath's life. Heath, living and breathing, coaching and preaching, is just as much of a miracle as Daniel was climbing out of the pit of lions.

The Casket

by Heath Williamson

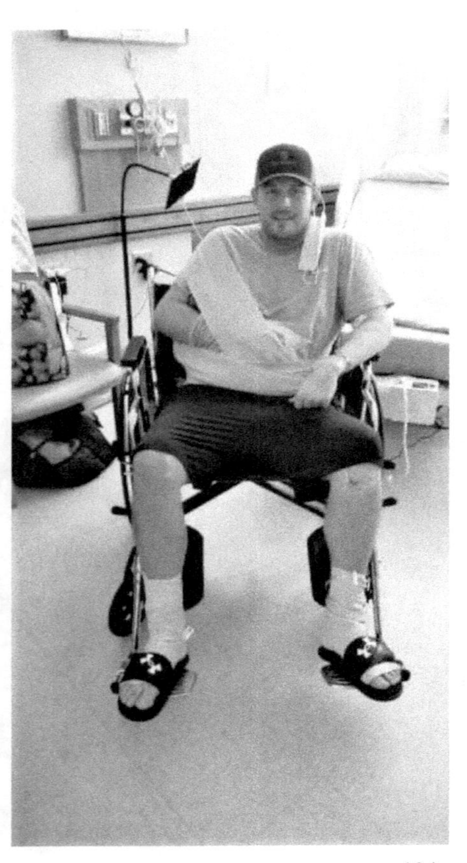

Only six days after coming home from our 77-day hospital stay, we made our first trip back to church. Rachel was adamant that it was too soon. Looking back, I can see how oblivious I was to all that she was dealing with emotionally. I felt such a strong burden to get back and see people that had loved, supported, and prayed for me. After parking around the back of the church, I slowly and gingerly eased inside the double doors of the church. At that point, it was still difficult for me to stand for any length of time, much less do much walking at all. So many familiar faces greeted us as we entered the sanctuary. Before the service began, we visited and cried with some of our closest friends and family.

As we sat down in the padded pew, everyone redirected their attention toward the front of the sanctuary. As I turned my attention toward the front as well, the Lord allowed me to see a vision or a glimpse. As plainly as I could have imagined, I saw a casket positioned in front of the church. It was light gray in color and it was trimmed in white. Sitting on top of the casket was a simple floral arrangement made of greenery mixed with several white and crimson flowers.

As I focused on the casket, it was made clear to me that it was my casket. Tears began to well up in my eyes. I could see Rachel with our six, beautiful children standing beside the casket as people were lined up to comfort them.

I sat there attempting to take in all that I was seeing. In those moments, it was as if the Lord Jesus himself spoke to me. *Heath, if it were not for me shielding you from the bulk of the electricity and choosing to spare your life, the next time you would have been in this church would have been in that casket.* Multiple doctors and nurses had already confirmed that truth many times, but there was a certain heaviness or gravity to what I experienced.

The Lord used this experience to remind me that every breath and every moment is a gift from Him. Every day we have an opportunity to bring honor and glory to the name of Jesus. And, what a blessing! After all, to serve and honor Jesus Christ is the reason for which we were all created, and it is the only way for us to be truly fulfilled. God has given you breath and life today. What are you doing with it?

Chapter 11
Confidence in the End

I lift up my eyes to the mountains –
where does my help come from?
My help comes from the Lord,
the maker of heaven and earth.
Psalm 121:1-2 (NIV)

This morning I awakened long before the sun began to peek over the horizon. I sit alone in the living room with numerous thoughts racing through my head in no particular order. Somehow, I feel much like I did morning after morning…evening after evening…surgery after surgery in that lonely hospital room. I waited day after day for vitals to be checked, longed impatiently week after week for answers and pleaded with the Lord to give me a sign that He was still there.

One thing I have learned through this journey is that the uneasiness in my mind and in my heart will never go away if I cannot get the thoughts out of my head, so I am currently putting them on paper. I have a strange, nauseated feeling that comes and goes over me. I randomly lose the desire to drink coffee, which I typically enjoy several cups of daily. A heavy tightness sits on my chest more times than not. There is an unexplained pain in my left jaw that has been a source of irritation since the third week in the hospital. I feel the emotions mounting on the inside, but I really have no idea how to release them. Tears never just come. I have taken more ibuprofen than I would like to admit to while dealing with a persistent headache, but I am reminded daily that this "trial" did not catch the Lord by surprise.

Because I really want the strangeness I feel to leave, I sometimes try to pretend like it is not really there. I wake up reminding myself not to carry it on the outside. The old saying about *walking in someone else's shoes* is so right. You cannot feel another person's hurt accurately unless you have been where they are. Friends have tried to remind me of truth as they attempt to sympathize. "You should be thankful," they will say. "Your husband is still alive." As I try to open up a tiny window of my heart to those around me, I am simply reminded to count my blessings. As true as this may be and as much as I have tried to lift high the name of the Lord even through this difficult time, I am asking the Lord to show me how to "practically" deal with the emotions I feel and I believe he is leading me.

I feel overwhelmed as I attempt to regain some type of structure in my home. Trying to retrain the younger children after being away from them for so long is hard. I realize the time with my older kids is shrinking and they will soon find their way out of my house. My ability to multi-task in my daily life has still yet to return to me. I have always been able to manage my household duties, exercise at some capacity, home-school my children, and get all 6 of them to the different places they needed to be, but my fine-tuned ability to multi-task is gone. And that can be quite frustrating for me at times.

I guess "Uncertainty" has made her home in my heart for now and she is producing fear and anxiety. Of course, I would like her to leave me alone and allow me to be reconciled in oneness with my husband, to reconnect with my children, and to catch up with friends that have loved me and prayed for me along this journey. But frequently, I must remind myself to simply breathe. I must focus on what is *real* for today. I must saturate my mind with the truth by reading God's Word. Some of the verses that are dearest to my heart, I now have hanging on the walls of my home so I can see them daily and be constantly reminded of where my focus should be even as my emotions come and go. These feelings that Uncertainty brings into my heart, however, are real. The emotions she causes to well up inside of me were created by the Creator himself. The struggles that I have, even in this moment, are not sinful in and of themselves, but it is important what I "do" with the emotions of the struggle. It is here where I hope to continue learning how to "apply" the wisdom and knowledge of God's Word and to share with you what He teaches me. It is the desire of God's heart that I focus on the blessings rather than dwelling on what seems to have been taken away.

Not long ago, we did a study on the different names of God. It was beyond beneficial for my spiritual life in the sense that it expanded my knowledge of God's character, who He is and what He is capable of. One of the names that we studied was the name *El Roi*, which means the *God who sees.* One of the main references in scripture that refers to this character of God is in the story of Hagar. Hagar was the handmaid of Sarai, Abraham's wife. Because Sarai was barren she gave Hagar to her husband, Abram, in hopes of having children through her. Of course, as soon as Hagar had the child, Sarai instantly began dealing harshly with her handmaid. Hagar did not ask to be put in the situation she was in. She did not expect to find herself pregnant with Abram's child. Hagar found herself in a difficult set of circumstances, but as we studied, the scripture says that Hagar called out to El Roi. She said in Genesis 16:13, You are the God that sees me.

As I pondered on Hagar and her situation, somehow, I could relate. As I dug further and further into God's Word, I felt the Lord speak to my heart. *I see you. I know your struggle. I know it is hard, but trust me. I am working out MY plan.* Something in my heart changed as I leaned on the Lord as El Roi. He could see my hurt, even when my family and friends could not see it. He could see that my heart wanted to be obedient, but I struggled to know what that looked like. When I looked at God my Father as El Roi, I began to feel almost as if He was walking by my side.

So often we are tempted to lie down and "wallow" – if that is even a word – in our situation. Speaking from personal experience, we like to talk about how bad things are, how unfairly we have been treated and how many things will have to fall into place by this certain time in order for other things to happen. We are finite in our thinking, because we cannot know the future. We feel the need to "know," but we struggle with trusting the Lord when we cannot see what He is trying to accomplish and yet, most of us would agree that we believe God knows what is best for us. So, why do we need to see and why do we need to be in control? Why is it hard for us to wait on the Lord to bring about His plans? The Lord *does not need us.* Sometimes He chooses to use people to bring about His plan, but He does not need us. He is omnipotent, meaning all-powerful, and He can make things fall into place exactly as He wishes, and He does not need any man to help Him do it. Goodness. If I could really get a handle on that truth alone, it could be absolutely life-changing! And yet…here I am again…trying to see, trying to be in control.

Tomorrow, we will be a year removed from the day of the accident. Thinking back to where I was a year ago brings back a flood of emotions I struggle to deal with. Although things in my marriage are significantly improved since our time in the hospital, I am still emotionally withdrawn from Heath at times. Often times, he is very much unaware of my struggle. As the days go by, I long for the proper feelings in my marriage to be restored to me. It is a tall order to act like my feelings as a wife are not different, especially in front of my children, who are extremely perceptive. It is difficult to talk about my struggle with Heath. He accurately remembers only a small amount from the day of the accident or the weeks and months that followed. He tries to empathize with how I might be feeling. I know however, it is unrealistic for me to ask him to understand my feelings, just as I could never accurately fathom all that he has been through this past year.

Recently, I began sharing small tidbits with Heath regarding my struggle. I have become fearful that my thoughts or feelings might get the best of me and I have realized that I could potentially succumb to the waywardness of my mind. The deepest desire of who I am absolutely loves Heath with every fiber of my being, but I am failing on a daily basis to convey that truth to him. My "feelings" for Heath occasionally come, but most often go. This is neither what I desire, nor what I know the Lord has for me to "feel." And yet, as most of us learned in marriage counseling, love is *not* a feeling. It is a *choice*. It is my job to *love* Heath regardless of whether or not I feel like it.

While I am working on my emotions and my heart, Heath is trying to regain as much physical strength and motion in his right hand as possible. Today, the therapy on his right hand and shoulder range of motion continues. Each week we work through new doctor's appointments and numerous physical evaluations. We should soon reach MMI, Maximum Medical Improvement. This is basically a formula used to determine the amount of Heath's disability. That concept alone is hard to swallow. So...this test and the percentage of disability that will follow him for the rest of his life, is based on a 4-hour test, conducted by someone who knows absolutely nothing about him. And this is what will shape the rest of our lives? Hmmm…something just seems pretty unfair about that concept altogether – and yet, that is what we are bound to because of the laws in the state of Alabama.

Although the accident my husband was involved in was not his fault, we have been advised by several legal counselors that there is nothing we can do to hold anyone accountable. Our lives as we knew them and the plans we had for our future have been changed forever. We are now expected to pick up the pieces and move on with our lives. This thought alone brings about an anger inside of me that I can honestly say, I have never felt before. It makes me want to bring about change and awareness. And yet, I must trust the Lord and believe what His word says. The "trial" I am going through did not catch Him by surprise and all the events of it passed through His hands.

There are days I feel that if I could "see" with my physical eyes that God was using all that we have been through for good, then it would be worth all the pain and the struggle. Or if he would just "write" with His finger on the wall so that my eyes could see, then maybe I would understand. Sometimes it all just feels wrong, so I want to do something to make it right. Something. Anything. I want answers. I need direction.

Sometimes I equally wish the voice of the Lord was audible. I wish my "ears" could actually hear His heart. But if I could, I would probably hear or see the Creator of the universe say or write something like this…

Why do you want to fix things? For me or for you? Why do you feel the deep need to expose the faults and failures of other people? Why do you feel the need to bring about justice? Is it for my glory? Or is it so that you can repay evil for evil? Why are you questioning the very One who breathed you into existence? Is it not I who knows all things?

111

For the last few weeks, I have been pleading with the Lord for answers. I have felt drawn to the story in the Bible about Joseph, the one who's brothers sold him into slavery and lied to their father about his death. I can see so much in Joseph's life that he must have deemed as "unfair." Surely, he looked up and asked the Lord, "why is all of this happening?" And yet, if you finish reading the story in the book of Genesis, God used Joseph to save the nation of Egypt as well as many people from other nations.

Once again, I felt like I could relate to him somehow. I felt like he had been mistreated or that people had wronged him. I can remember pleading with the Lord for direction and for answers almost in anger. I would pray, *What about Potiphar's wife!?!* How could she get away with forcing herself on an innocent man and then lying to have him thrown in prison. *What about Joseph's brothers!?!* They sold Joseph into slavery and then lied to their father saying that wild animals killed their brother. *Is there NO RECORD of justice being brought about?* I studied. I cross-referenced. I pleaded with the Lord to show me my heart as He saw it. I struggled to understand. I was broken…hurt…angry…bitter…frustrated…and confused. I guess I questioned the Lord, day in and day out for a couple of weeks…*what are you trying to accomplish? What is the plan? Lord, surely this is not the way you will bring yourself honor and glorify your name.*

But…He answered me. My heart was genuinely calling out to Him and after weeks of seeking His heart, He answered me. Late one evening when I was at my breaking point, I was scurrying around…decorating tables for a home-school event…tears pouring down my face…all alone…and I asked the Lord out loud, *was Joseph's pain and suffering ever justified!?!* And the Lord led me that night, through my pastor, to Genesis 50:19-21. It was simple. The answers to my questions were right there in the scripture in black and white. The verse read, "And Joseph said to them, do not be afraid, am I in the place of God?" Joseph chose to forgive. He chose to leave the outcome up to God. He refused to dwell in all that was unfair.

Let me take you back and refresh your memory on where we find Joseph at this point in his life. Joseph's brothers hated him to the point they contemplated killing him by throwing him into a deep well. Then, they collectively decided it would be more profitable for them to sell their brother and make some money, so they sold him into slavery to the Egyptians. He was separated from his father and mother and the life he had always known…for no good reason. And yet through God's blessing on his life, Joseph found himself second in command in the nation of Egypt. Only the king himself was more powerful than Joseph. And God used all the unfair circumstances in Joseph's life to bring about salvation for the human race. Sure. Joseph could have pitched a fit. He could have resisted. But rather he submitted to the Lord and was willing to be used for the glory of God.

Why do I say all of these things? Why do I allow my heart to reflect on my past? Why do I paint the picture of it for you? Why do I take the time to open the curtains to my glass house, so you can see all the yucky thoughts that go through my mind? It is simple. So that you can see that I am real. My situation is real. My mind is real. My hurt is real. My struggles are real. My family is real. And so that you can be assured that I know you are real. Your struggles may be different from mine, but they are real. Your hurt is real. There may not be anyone else that can understand your pain or know your struggle, but that does not change that it is real. The question is though: how are *you* dealing with the pain…the hurt…the loss…the struggle?? Are you allowing yourself to be buried in the hurt or are you choosing to take it before the Lord?

Multiple times a day I think about this scripture that was so dear to me in the hospital that I wrote it on the mirror in the bathroom. It comes from the book of Philippians (4:6) and it says, "Do not be anxious about anything, but in everything, by prayer and petition, *with thanksgiving,* present your requests to God." So many times, we stop reading there. But if you continue to read the following verse, it says this: "And the peace of God, which transcends all understanding, will guard your hearts and minds in Christ Jesus." *Peace?* Yeah…that is what I need when my chest is so tight, I have to remind myself to breathe. *Which transcends all understanding?* Meaning I *can* have peace even when I don't understand? Yes. That is what the Word of God teaches. But…how often do I *actually* stop what I am doing…thank the Lord…and then ask Him to intervene. If I want the peace that goes beyond what I can understand, it requires action on my part and the Lord is continuing to teach me how to do that practically.

Even as I find myself in the midst of this trial that seems like it may never end, I am reminded when James tells us to "consider it pure joy, my brethren, *when* you face trials of many kinds" (James 1:2). He does not say *if* you face trials, but *when.* He goes on to say that "the testing of your faith develops perseverance" (James 1:3). Sheeeew! So today, even as I continue through this current trial, I can be assured that this will NOT be the last hardship that will come my way. And I believe that this verse is helping us to see that the trial itself can be for our own good. We CAN profit from the struggle. The difficult times can not only be a time of learning how to persevere, but it can also be a time where the Lord prepares us for what is to come. The God that created us is omniscient. He is all-knowing and He knows what is to come. He also knows our hearts and what we need. And He is capable of bringing those things about WITHOUT our help. Therefore, He can always be trusted.

Behind the Mask

By: Maddie Williamson

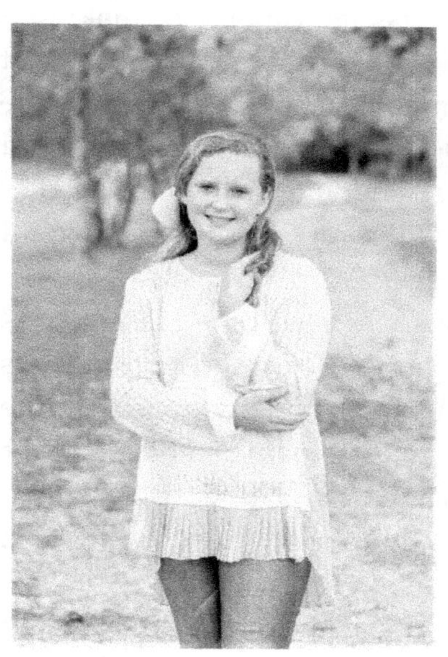

I grew up very quickly the day that Mom dropped me off at my aunt's house on her way to the hospital to see Daddy. I remember like it was yesterday, climbing out of our light grey Suburban, with my 5 siblings. We were unsure, scared and confused. I remember how Mom seemed so sure that everything would be fine and even as tears fell from her face, she had a deep hope in the Lord. She was confident that He would show us the way.

Once we were all safe inside the house, I can remember still feeling scared, but like I needed to hold how I felt inside. I was not used to the overwhelming emotions that I felt that day. I had always been really good at keeping my emotions put together. Even if I was a mess on the inside, I have always been able to keep the outside clean and pretty. I did not want anyone to see the ugly mess that I felt like I was. I especially did not want my siblings to see me afraid. Honestly, I did not even want to admit to myself how I felt. I wanted to be strong and solid for my siblings. As the oldest, I wanted to be the one they could hold onto as everything seemed to fall apart around us.

Alone, I walked out onto the carport once I realized I could no longer hold the tears back. I will never forget remembering the words mom spoke to us before she drove away. "I love you and it is going to be ok," she said before pulling out of the driveway. Little did I know that neither she, nor Dad, would be home for the next 3 months. Our family was being pulled apart at the seams.

I would soon find out that I was *not* capable of making it alright. That no amount of singing could fix everything, but that God was the only one who could hold us together. He was the only source of hope. Even though we were afraid, we would need to look to the Lord as our stronghold. He would need to be our strength. He would be the solid rock to which we would cling, while life seemed to collapse.

Just like I have heard daddy share each time He gives his testimony of the accident, "My hope is built on nothing less than Jesus' blood and righteousness...I dare not trust the sweetest frame, but wholly lean on Jesus' name." I have known the words to that hymn since I was 7 years old, but suddenly it made sense. If our hope is on anything other than Jesus Christ and his righteousness, we have missed the mark!

Since the day of the accident, I have had a hard time feeling emotions again. Mom and I have often used the analogy of being a 2-liter bottle that has been filled with our emotions since the day of Dad's accident. Suddenly, one day my bottle was violently shaken. The cap of the bottle was loosened by a memory. As the cap came off the bottle, the contents that had been so neatly kept inside, were uncontrollably being spilled out all over the floor.

In the past, even in the midst of hard times, I have always been able to put on a "fake" face. I have been able to act like everything is ok, when in reality, it is far from "ok." Like with everything, the longer I practiced, the better I got at "acting." After years of wearing the "mask", I had begun to wear it very well.

I have always liked being in control, but this was a situation that I really had no control over! I was at the Lord's mercy. I was no longer in the "driver's seat." It was time for me to sit back and see what God had in store for our family.

After Daddy's accident, I have had a hard time being "real." I have struggled dealing with all of the emotions that I poured into my bottle. During our time without Mom and Dad, my bottle exploded at random times. Those that happened to be around as the explosion took place saw the Maddie that is not always "pretty and in order", but it was the "real" me. I have had to get used to letting other people see beyond the fake mask that I have embraced so well in the past.

Being "real" has most definitely been a struggle for me, but God has been teaching me to trust Him. Psalms 40: 8 tells us, "I delight to do your will, O my God, and your law is within my heart." Those words pierce me. I had the "obeying" part down. But the "delighting" was hard. For me, I felt more like one of the pharisees clanking their tithes into the offering plate. My life was just a show.

Shortly after Dad was discharged, I heard *The Stained-Glass Masquerade* by Casting Crowns. I could identify with the words of that song. It was a picture of me so many times…feeling the tug of the Spirit but being a little bit too proud to admit that there were things that needed addressing. It described my life as I tried to hide behind all of my circumstances. I could identify with the phrase, "Only when no one is watching, can we really fall apart." It spoke to my heart and showed me that there are times when life is hard, but it is ok to let other people see the struggle! The very next line of the song says, "but would it set me free...if I dared to let you see...the truth behind the person...that you've imagined me to be?"

I began asking myself questions. Would it be encouraging to someone else if they knew the real me? Would people be encouraged if they could see that other people had issues? If they could see that a believers' life is sometimes messy and we are often scattered?

God has taught me that even in difficult times, He loves each one of us and He has a plan. He is bringing about the plan for our good! I want to be able to live my life being real with myself and with the Lord. I want to be able to live in the glass house. I want others to see that God is good and no matter how difficult the circumstances, He is able to use us for HIS glory, regardless of how crazy and scattered as we may be. It is through our weakness His power can be put on display!

Chapter 12
Scars

For the eyes of the Lord run to and fro throughout
the whole earth, seeking to show himself strong
on behalf of those whose heart is loyal to Him.
2 Chronicles 16:9

Looking back to our months in the hospital, I had all of my natural healing remedies, herbal teas, and essential oils in our hospital room right alongside the medication Heath was being given. I guess I felt like I was helping somehow, and I did to some degree. Because I have seasonal allergies, some days the lemon, lavender, and peppermint essential oils diffusing from our room could be smelled all the way down the hall of the 6th floor. On other days I had a blend of calming or uplifting oils diffusing to help with whatever mood in which I found myself that day.

Lavender would most likely be considered by most people in the "oily community" to be the most versatile essential oil and we use it daily in our home for anything from bug bites and allergies to calming roll-on blends and burns. According to my research, while I was in the hospital, it was suggested by many to be very effective in reducing the outward appearance of scaring. So…of course – I gathered all of the oils and resources

I had in that hospital room and created a plan to "help" Heath with all of the "scars" that he was certain to have.

I remember like it was yesterday, climbing into the hospital bed with him and explaining all I had learned in my hours of research. He listened, but after I finished my spill, he calmly said, "No. I want to see the scars. As ugly as they will be, they will be a reminder of what God has done for me. For us. For our family. These scars will be an Ebenezer of God's faithfulness to us."

I was stunned. I thought to myself, *seriously? You don't even want to try? You will have several deep scars. They are going to be big and really dark and no oil I have is good enough to make them go completely away…maybe just lessen the appearance.*

Hearing what he said to me that day was not easy to hear, but I have gone back to it time and time again. The tragic accident Heath went through was *not* for nothing and the wounds he had would eventually heal completely. Time would allow his body to mend and all that would remain were the scars. Although his physical body will be changed forever, God can still use the scars of his body to remind people of what He is capable of doing. I understood the truth, but I still felt empty. I was thankful for his perspective and aware of God's goodness. I was proud of Heath that he could even have such a positive outlook in the depth of his situation, but I longed for healing as well.

It was during the study on the names of God we looked at a few months back that I remember hearing the name *Jehovah Rapha*. This name refers to the name of God meaning *the God who heals*. The Lord spoke to my heart during the study and my prayer time following it. He opened my eyes to who He really is. Our God is capable of healing me, too. Emotionally. Physically. Intimately. Spiritually. Not only does He see where I am, as He saw Hagar, but He can bring about the healing I have been longing for and searching to find.

The last few months have been challenging for me to say the least, in the sense that from all outsiders looking in, Heath is "healed." The doctors have released him to go back to work. The test has been run to tell him how "disabled" he is. So basically, from a physical standpoint, he is as good as he will get. While I can honestly say that I am so thankful for his healing, there are more times than not that I still feel like the wounds of my heart are in many ways so fresh. Raw. Open. Vulnerable to the lies of the enemy.

If I am honest, there are days that I wish Heath would leave me and take the kids. Not leave me for another woman or even out of spite, but because I love him and I want so desperately for him to be able to put all of the last 15 months behind him and strive to be all that God is calling him to be. The enemy knows our weakest points and he plants seeds in our minds and so often we allow them to take root. How many times I have thought, *Heath does not deserve to have all the extra baggage that my heart is causing? He should not have to deal with all of my issues in addition to all that he has already had to endure.*

But that is a lie. Heath's first calling is to be my leader...my rock...my head. If I measure my thought of Heath leaving me up to the "plumb line" of the word of God, I KNOW that my thought is disobedient. It is in no way a part of God's perfect plan for me. Or for Heath. Or for our children. Or for our church. Or for our community. Therefore, I should take that thought captive and not allow it to take root in my heart. And I should equally take measures to allow others to hold me accountable.

If I will allow myself to be truthful, I have contemplated going away for a time myself. Not using the word "divorce," just for a period of time. Though never vocalized until last week (so that I could be held accountable), I have pondered, *that maybe a short time of separation would be good for us. Maybe without the kids, it would allow me to pray and seek the Lord more fervently. And if the Lord shows us that we could heal more quickly apart, then the separation would be easier. The poor kids would not have to see me struggle every day and I would not be a reminder to them of how hard things have been. They too would heal more quickly.* Sounds plausible...right??? *We love each other too much to stay together and it would be easier to go separate ways. Being together brings out the hurt and I want to put this behind us and move on.* Sounds pretty convincing...huh?? Maybe you have even found yourself right where I have been.

Can you see how the deceiver works? Satan knows how to weasel his way into your heart! These thoughts that were so real, yet difficult to write down, are straight from the pit of hell. They are exactly what the enemy is hoping to accomplish. He wants to tear our family apart from the inside out. He does not need drugs and alcohol to do it. He does not need adultery. He can simply plant a seed of doubt that completely undermines the nature of what God has created us to be.

Heath and I vowed before the Lord on September 2, 2006, to remain together for better or worse...in sickness and in health...for rich or for poor. These past several months have certainly not been the *better* of our 15 years together. There has certainly been more *sickness* than good health. And despite what everyone in our small community thinks, there has been no huge settlement due to Heath's accident that has made us rich. But God's word is clear. I should stay.

The other night I had a dream that I know was from the Lord. Honestly, I remember very little from the dream itself, but I understood the meaning of it. It was as if God himself "visibly" showed me that Satan had planted the lie in my heart. He helped me to see that a tragedy in a person's life can quickly turn their thoughts to a very dark and sinful place if they do not actively fight against the evil one. The scripture says "he comes to steal, kill, and destroy."

The desire of Satan, the enemy himself, is that I be alone. He desires to steal my children's hearts and minds through what they hear and what they see at school. He wants to steal their innocence with the small electronic devices that everyone now has in their purse or pocket. He wants to kill my marriage. He wants to destroy my family, because he knows that God's plan is best for me. He knows that it will be more difficult for others to see the glory of the Lord if he can succeed in tearing our family apart.

There are times when you and I can make valid arguments in our minds, but we *must* run from the lies. We cannot entertain these thoughts from the deceiver himself. We must not wallow in our situations, but rather get up and fight for what God has so richly blessed us with. We must be encouraged to fight for our marriages and the hearts of our children. As ironic as it seems, we must actively fight for peace in the storms of life so that we may not be overcome by the lies of Satan while we are in the valley.

What has made us believe today that we should never hurt? Why are we conditioned to think we should never feel pain? What has made us think that if we go through difficult times, we should just bail or throw in the towel? The path of obedience is never easy, but it is the only way to true fulfillment. It is the way God designed us to live; therefore, it is perfect. And even as I am continuing to understand these truths on a personal level, the Lord reminds me to look to Him. He knows the way to life everlasting. The things that I long to encourage you with today have not been easy for me to live by recently.

Often, I have tried to put into words what I have dealt with or how I have felt deep in the core of who I am. Maybe the best word to use is "numbness." I just felt nothing. I had closed my heart completely so that I would feel nothing at all. Not feelings of happiness...sadness...frustration...anger...or hurt.

Nothing...really. Things happened daily that would typically get me up out of my seat, but after the accident, I had quite a few periods of time where nothing phased me.

The feeling of numbness to the world around me might be better explained as just a feeling of indifference. I had no desire to fight for my marriage...to train up my children in the fear and admonition of the Lord...to clean and reorganize my house...to be one with my husband...to socialize or interact with people at all. But...I believe that the Lord is answering me as I continue to plead with Him for practical answers.

I have questioned my relationship with the Lord...questioned my marriage...questioned my identity as a believer...and even questioned my life in general. But God has *always* confirmed His love for me. He would send a word through a friend or allow me to hear a song or something completely irrelevant to my situation that would be a simple reminder to me that El Roi saw me. And I knew in my heart of hearts that He was in control, even when I felt completely out of control. My *only* hope was to turn to Him.

There have been several times that I have been at a very, very low point since Heath's accident. Every person that I talked to encouraged me to go get help. Numerous people offered stories of their own personal testimonies of different medications that would uplift my spirits. Three specific times I stood in my bedroom alone. The feeling of hopelessness consumed me. I dug the bottle out of the bottom of Heath's drawer and held it in my hand. It was legal. I had a prescription for it. And I just wanted to escape. I wanted to be kind to my family and to love them the way they deserved to be loved. But as I stood holding the bottle, I heard the Lord speak so loudly to my heart that it had to be audible. *I am enough. I am enough, Rachel. You have taken your eyes off of me and you are trying to fix it in your strength. I am enough. Do you trust me? Do you trust that I am enough?*

Maybe the Lord had been sheltering me somehow by not allowing me to "feel" the pain. Maybe the dream I had a few nights ago was the wake-up call I needed. Either way, if I trust the Lord, I have to believe that He was working the best for me, even if I cannot see it. I was in the darkest place I have ever been in my life and yet, the Lord whispered to my heart that *He was enough.* And yes, you guessed. I put the bottle back in the drawer, picked up my Bible and my journal, and began to pray for practical answers.

Why do I feel the freedom to share these things with you? Why have I opened up my heart and allowed you to see the ugliness? Again, the answer is quite simple. I want you to know that God is real. Am I trying to say that no one should ever take medication? Of course not! My husband took so much medication in the hospital that it made my head spin. The main focus here is that God can help us if we will allow Him the opportunity. I want you to believe that He can reach down and touch your life wherever you find yourself. Regardless of whether you appear to have it all together or your life is in shambles as mine was, God can pull you out of the pit.

As I have mentioned several times, I have pleaded with the Lord for direction, and I ultimately felt the leading to write this book for my healing. And as it has filled the blank pages of a white 3-ring binder, I have found freedom. As only God can do, He has given me the freedom to hurt. The freedom to cry. The freedom to be vulnerable. The freedom to admit the anger. The freedom to express what is really in my heart, so that I can ultimately be "freed" from it.

Again, I ask you as I ask myself: Why are we conditioned to think we should never "feel" bad things? What makes us think that we should never hurt or feel pain? Maybe it is simply because in the world we live in today it is so easy to mask it. To run from it. To hide behind it. Or maybe because it is just easier to bury the hurt than to deal with the pain. Most of us have been there at some point or another in life. And I would wager if you have been, you would most likely agree that the wound never really fully heals if it is not dealt with.

At one point after coming home from the hospital, I remember sitting with Heath in a session with our Christian counselor and trying to express what my feelings were to him. He was patient and very well versed in God's word. The best analogy I could come up with was this: I said to him, "I feel like a 2-liter bottle. I have been pouring emotions into the bottle for the last several months. Now that we are back home, trying to get back to life as normal, I feel like the 2-liter bottle has been violently shaken and I need someone to take the lid off to release the pressure. The counselor assured me that as I continued to look to the Lord, the time for healing would come. He prayed for us before every meeting. He assured me that it was okay to cry. It was okay to hurt. The feelings I had were not a lack of trust in the Lord, but that God was able to heal my heart and restore me to Heath again.

It has taken me a while to understand exactly what he meant, but over the last several weeks, I am beginning to understand. Just as Heath has physical scars that have changed who he is, I too will have scars – emotional scars. The bottoms of both Heath's feet, the back of his right leg, his thigh, his stomach, and his right arm/hand will remind him forever of God's goodness; therefore, he has embraced the scars. They are now a part of the man that he is.

In some ways, I see the writing of this book as an opportunity to outwardly express the inward pain and hurt I have experienced. Just as Heath has been changed by the traumatic event, I too will be changed through it. Scarred, if you will. Emotionally scarred. But, once the wounds of my heart fully heal, and with time and the Lord's continued help, I believe they will, I want the pages of this book to be an outward reflection of my inner scars. I want to look through these pages and see the words of my heart poured out. I want this book to be an "Ebenezer" for me, just as the 12 stones from the middle of the Jordan River were for the Israelites in the book of Joshua. I want to embrace the scars…the change…the growth…and be forever grateful that God has brought about this time in my life. I want to be thankful that He was with me through it all. Rather than continuing to "live" in the hurt of the past, I want to strive to be used by the Lord and to bring honor and glory to His great name.

Rather than trying to "go back" to what life once was, I want to embrace all that God has brought us through and look for opportunities to "use" all that we have learned. I want to remember how real it was and how the Lord carried me. Each day I live, I want to be able to look back on this season of my life and be reminded of my spiritual growth and deep dependence on the Lord for my strength.

My hope for you as you close the pages of this book, place it on the shelf in your room, or share it with a friend is that you will be encouraged. This life is not one that we should strive to live alone. Scripture is clear that we are not to "forsake the assembling of ourselves together." We need other believers to speak truth into our lives. We need to hear the stories of other believers who also can testify to the faithfulness of our God.

I want you to be reminded of the scripture in 2 Chronicles 16:9 that says "the eyes of the Lord roam to and fro, seeking to show Himself strong on behalf of those whose hearts are turned towards Him." He wants us to share our stories. He does not want us to keep it all buried inside. He wants to work miracles on our behalf so that He can show himself strong through us.

He wants us to see our struggles as an opportunity to grow in our knowledge and understanding of who He really is. He desires that we look to Him for answers and that we praise His name from the rooftops when he responds.

The emotions – of pain…of hurt…of anger…of betrayal…of loss – are not sinful emotions and we should not believe the lie of Satan that they are. It is what we *do* with those emotions that can be harmful to us or get us in trouble. Rather than "wallowing" in our situation…the hurt…the pain…the anger…the betrayal…the loss, we must *choose* to *actively* take it to the Lord. It is not a passive action. It is actively searching for strength from the Lord to "take our thoughts captive," refusing to dwell on the negative, but rather choosing to take our situation before our Heavenly Father and ask Him to draw near to us as we draw near to Him. In your struggle, refuse to turn to worldly things that will simply help you escape reality and mask your pain. Get to the source.

It was only 3 days after coming home from the hospital that Heath was alone in the living room, praying and seeking the Lord about all that had gone on in our lives. He heard a song that came through the Bluetooth speaker on top of the white, antique armoire next to the couch. He felt the Lord speak to his heart as he heard a short excerpt from John Piper in the song "Though You Slay Me," by Shane and Shane.

The message was that everything we go through in life is not meaningless. If we are following the Lord in obedience, all that we go through in this life is for a purpose. We must focus on the eternal. We may never understand all that God is doing on this side of heaven, but we must trust that he has a plan.

This truth has been life-changing for me. It requires action. It means focused and intentional choices to keep from losing sight of the eternal goal. If you have trusted the Lord as your Savior, be encouraged. Take heart. Do not quit. The world is in desperate need and we are called to love others. Do not live in fear, but rather seek out people to bless and share the love of Christ with them. There is no greater calling in this life.

When you are on the mountains of life, commit God's word to memory. Hide the truth, from the very One who spoke you into existence, deep inside the core of who you are. Saturate your mind with pure and holy, knowing that the valleys of life are often deep and lengthy, but that God is capable of bringing back those truths to encourage your heart when you need it the most.

It is possible to go through struggles and hardships while allowing your heart to sing with confidence. We must not look to what is seen, but to what is unseen. Day by day, put the negative out of your mind. Do not allow it to stay. Focus on a simple truth from God's word, rather than inspirational speakers who just help you feel better. Write the truths down. Put them on your mirror. Tape a note card to the dash in your car. Remove obstacles that hinder your focus. *Choose you this day whom you will serve.*

As I leave this collection of thoughts from my brain with you, I desperately want you to feel the same peace from the Holy Spirit that I have felt for years as I have walked with the Lord, but especially in the last 10 months where he has vividly allowed me to see His hand. My prayer for you is that the Lord meets you exactly where you are. He knows your past. He knows your hurts and your failures. He understands your emotional highs and lows. He sees the anger that is buried so deeply within you that you forgot it was there. But – He longs to show you the way. He wants to fulfill you as you look to Him.

Be encouraged today for you still have this life to live, so make the most of it. We can be certain that the trials will come, but ponder the words from the songwriter, Louis Kathman: "Why do I sail my ship in a spoonful of water, knowing life is a vapor and eternity is a sea?" We must be eternally minded, knowing that this earthly life we live is not all there is. Call out to the Lord wherever you find yourself. Ask Him to meet you where you are. Choose gratitude – every day. Resist the devil and he will flee from you.

The final thought I will leave you with is a verse that I clung to while we were in the hospital. It was short and simple, but it is powerful:

"Return to your rest, O my soul,
For the LORD has dealt bountifully with you."
Psalm 116:7

Just a Nobody

By Heath Williamson

As I was lying in the hospital a few days after the accident, I found myself pondering why God would save my life. I am so thankful that years ago God made me aware of my sin and my need of forgiveness. At nine years old, I believed and trusted in the love that God has shown to the whole world through Christ Jesus. My salvation and my eternity are secure because Jesus Christ paid the price for my sin - a price that I could never pay.

I know that had I died on the day of the accident, 75-feet in the air, that I would have opened my eyes in the presence of the Lord. Although I am far from perfect, God did not save my life to give me another chance to be right with Him. I am confident that God spared my life to give me a chance to live every day for Him with a sense of urgency.

The Bible says that if the gospel is hidden that it is hidden from the lost. That is my purpose. I want to honor God in every role in which He has placed me. I want to be the kind of husband for Rachel that God has called me to be. Marriage is an absolute blessing from God and I am always amazed at how fulfilling it is when we seek to do things the way He has instructed us to. God is wise and His ways are perfect.

I want to be "daddy" to my kids. I want to be the kind of daddy that loves them enough to lead and point them to the

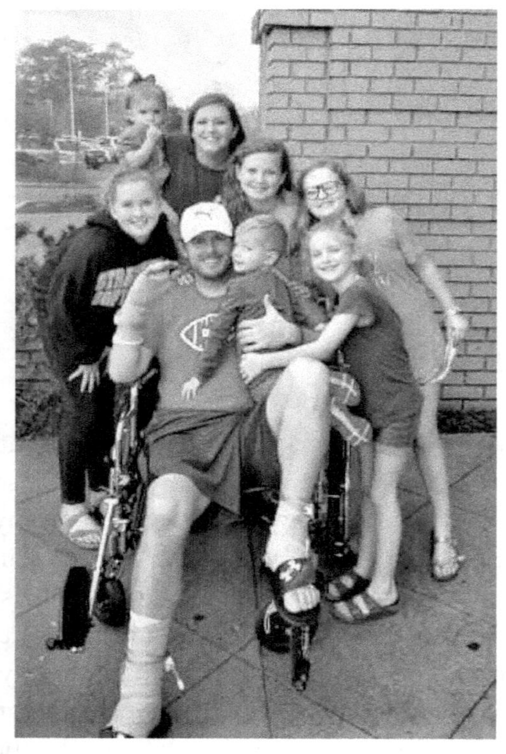

Lord. I want to live out God's design for my children every single day, giving God an opportunity to show Himself strong and faithful. I want to share the hope that we have in the gospel of Jesus Christ, in whatever capacity God chooses to allow me.

Closing my eyes in what I thought was certain death, and God choosing to spare my life has given me a better understanding of what the apostle Paul meant when he said "for me to live is Christ, and to die is gain." Every day that we live here on this earth is an opportunity to worship and bring honor to the name of our Lord and Savior, Jesus Christ. So, until the Lord calls me home - I'm just a nobody...trying to tell everybody...all about somebody...who saved my soul.

Epilogue

As I think back on Heath's accident and the miracle that he is walking through my house every day, I cannot help but think back to my life before him and of the "miracle" it is that we even found each other in the beginning. I think about the events the Lord orchestrated to bring us together, and yet, I am reminded of the painful process and how God grew me through that time. Just last week I heard a quote, "Don't ever get comfortable with being comfortable. It is in the discomfort that growth takes place."

Those words have most definitely been true in my life. The hard times...the struggles...the pain...the heartache...the uncertainty...the abandonment...the loneliness...the fear. While we travel through the hard and uncomfortable times on this journey we call "life," we can certainly grow, but only *if* we can find it in ourselves to look to the One who knows our deepest needs.

Acknowledgements

I want to acknowledge first and foremost, my Lord and Savior, Jesus Christ for walking with me through the darkest days of my life. I experienced the love and faithfulness of the Lord in a way that will forever mark me.

Heath, my husband and best-friend - you have more strength than any man alive and you are the rock on which I lean. You have steadied my wavering heart and you always point me back to the cross. You always help remind me of what we were created for. Thank you for loving me through the good times as well as the bad and even the really ugly. I am so proud of the man you are and so thankful to call you mine. I love you.

My 6 beautiful children - you are resilient, strong and courageous. You have upheld me and encouraged me as I struggled after daddy's accident. You will never know what you mean to me. Thank you for helping me stay afloat with all the dishes and laundry. Thank you for the cards and notes of encouragement. I love all 6 of you.

Michael and Cristin Murphy, our forever friends – There are few days that go by without me thinking of you. I so desperately wish that you had not had to travel this road with us. Michael – You are an inspiration to all. You are such a fighter and I am beyond proud of you. No one can keep a good man down. Cristin – I could not have made it without you. You are a great wife and a blessing to Michael. I am so proud of your attitude and all you have taken on after this accident changed our lives. We may never fully understand why all of this happened to us, but with the Lord's help, we survived "the hospital" together. Thank you for everything.

The nursing staff at USA hospital in Mobile, AL. - You were amazing, and the Lord blessed me through you.

Dr. Bright and Dr. Butts – You fought for my husband and loved me along the way. I will forever be grateful for you.

Dr. McKee and Dr. Burkett – You came together and saved Heath's right hand. I often think of you when I see it. Thank you for allowing the Lord to use you.

Dr. Thornton – Thank you for the funny stories to brighten the really hard days and for the burrito surprise.

Mike and Joan Eubanks, my 2nd parents – Words cannot describe my gratefulness for you. You held me when I needed comfort and reminded me of scripture when my heart began to doubt. You allowed your home to be a place of refuge for me during the countless surgeries Heath had. You prayed over me when I could not find words to pray on my own, and you lifted me up when I began to crumble under the pressure. You will forever have a special place in my heart. I love you guys.

Rooted and Grounded, a coffee shop in Mobile, AL – I was covered by God's Word in your coffee shop. God used you to keep me from dwelling on the bad. He encouraged my spirit through the scriptures on the walls and the music played in the shop. Thank you.

Richard and Nancy Cochran, my parents – for allowing your home to be home to my children for 3 months. I know it is a tall order to go from <u>no</u> children at home to having a house full of kids, but you did it. I love you.

Roger and Tammy Cochran, my aunt and uncle and Tiffany, my cousin – Thank you for meeting my practical needs and for staying on your knees in prayer for me. Thanks for the Mexican food, the stamps, the numerous copies and the washed clothes. You blessed me beyond measure.

Good News Baptist Chapel Fellowship – I will not try to name all of the blessings from your fellowship. From the work you did at our house and keeping up the yard to the prayers, encouragement and visits, I will forever be grateful. Each one of you is a tremendous blessing from the Lord.

Mike and Cindy Williamson, Heath's parents – Thank you for loving me and accepting me as your family. Thank you for supporting the kids while we were away and helping them get from one place to another. I love you both.

Caleb and Abby, my brother and sister-in-law – Thank you for giving me your car to use for 3 months. It was such a blessing and saved me a ton on gas. Thank you also for helping with my children and being there to talk when they needed you.

Andrea and Andrew, my sister and brother-in-law – Thank you for opening your home and allowing me to leave my kids with you at a moment's notice. Thank you for the practical help at my house and for checking time-sensitive things off my to-do list.

Line-crew co-workers – You are like brothers to Heath. There are no words for the way you rallied around my husband and encouraged my soul with funny stories and memories of Heath. I will never forget the feeling I had when I pulled into the parking lot of the hospital to see all of you, along with your wives, standing together as one. It was overwhelming. Thank you for everything.

Dr. Richard Atwell, counselor at New Life Counseling – God absolutely sent us to you. Thank you for knowing scripture to combat each one of my fears and doubts. Thank you for helping me to realize that emotions are not sinful and for helping me trust the Lord through all my doubts and fears. I am forever grateful for our time together.

Nancy Wiggins – thank you for being honest and truthful with me and for making suggestions that made this book easier to understand and follow. I appreciate your willingness to help me with this book and your persistence in telling me "what a good catch Heath would be."

Wesley Jeffcoat – thank you for allowing your office to be my office as I wrote this book. The hours I spent in front of your computer allowed my handwritten pages to become legible and printable. You have also been an encouragement and mentor to me for over 15 years. Thank you for your willingness to pray for me and invest in me.

Paul and Eugene, P & L Publishing and Literary Services – You have been such a blessing to me. Thank you from the bottom of my heart for your patience with me and for helping me put "our story" in the form of a book. God has certainly gifted you both and I am beyond grateful for your professional suggestions and godly perspectives. Thanks a million!

The Bluebird Coffee Company in Andalusia – thank you for allowing me to use the couch by the fire and the free wi-fi. Your business has been a blessing to so many.

My story would not be complete without acknowledging all the people of our community and even co-ops all over the southeast for your generous support and prayers for our family. Often times, people like to focus on how bad things are, but we have seen the good in people and are eternally grateful for those that allowed the Lord to use them in our times of greatest need. We have prayed that the Lord would bless you for your love and care for us. Thank you from the bottom of my heart.

www.ingramcontent.com/pod-product-compliance
Lightning Source LLC
Chambersburg PA
CBHW061303120726
48001CB00001B/456